CRAIG

The Boy Who Lives

NEVILLE SEXTON ～

Gill & Macmillan

Gill & Macmillan Ltd
Hume Avenue, Park West, Dublin 12
with associated companies throughout the world
www.gillmacmillan.ie

© Neville Sexton 2011
978 07171 4862 2

Design and print origination by Carole Lynch
Printed by Scandbook AB, Sweden

This book is typeset in Quadraat and
Stone Sans.

The paper used in this book comes from the wood
pulp of managed forests. For every tree felled, at least
one tree is planted, thereby renewing natural
resources.

A CIP catalogue record for this book is available from
the British Library.

5 4 3 2 1

'This book is a harrowing account of every parent's nightmare. Brutally honest and revealing, Neville Sexton's extraordinary telling of his story is a must read.'

Daniel McConnell, Sunday Independent

'A remarkable story of a remarkable family that takes us on a journey that spans most of the emotions of life—joy, happiness, terrible sorrow and loss. But most of all it's a story of the enduring power of the human spirit and of sheer, never-give-up love. Neville Sexton's moving tribute to his son Craig is also testament to all the other families down the years who have gone through the same life-changing experience.'

Tim O'Connor, former Secretary General to the President

'A true and powerful story of a boy whose love never died.'

Rasher (aka Mark Kavanagh), Irish contemporary artist

For You, Craig

All that you were, you remain.
And so much more ...

CONTENTS

His breath is the hush of gentle winds that swirl in sleepy,
meadowed glens
That blow the thistle-down to sky, that whisper softly
'I'm Alive'
And though winter stole Him from our sight to bring Him
to forever light
To somewhere that we cannot know—He still leaves
footprints in the snow

ACKNOWLEDGEMENTS

We'd like to take this opportunity to say thanks to a number of very special people who have, in one way or another, given their support to us.

When Craig first got sick Barbara and I left our jobs to spend all of our time with him. We cannot quantify the eternal gratitude that we hold in our hearts for the generosity, the very best of humanity, extended to us by those we knew, those we worked with and the many we'll never know. So to all the staff in Galileo Ireland, BT Ireland, Trinity Biotech, the many Travel Agents around the country and those who lent their support we are so deeply thankful. The financial aid given allowed us the peace of mind and freedom to just be with our son through the darkest and also most powerful moments of his life. There are of course individual people who deserve particular thanks for this but at the risk of leaving someone out all we'll say is this: You know who you are, and we'll never forget what you did.

When it came to getting this book published there are a few people we wish to single out for particular thanks:

To my little sister Melanie. I cannot thank you enough for putting me, and the book, in contact with some very important people. Maybe one day, and I don't know how, I can put you in contact with a certain Robert Pattinson . . . ye just never know, Mel!

To an old school friend, Alan Prendergast (that's 'Prendo' to those of us in the know), whose father died only weeks after Craig. We want to say a special thanks for the support, the energy and the contacts you gave to help get Craig's book noticed by the publishing world. We appreciate the special efforts you made on our behalf.

To Rasher (whom I know from school but everyone else knows as a world famous artist). I want to say thanks for reading and lending your name and comment to the book.

To Marianne Gunn O'Connor for encouraging me to write this book in the first place and for allowing me to believe that it could be published. We are so grateful for that push and for putting us in contact with the agents who eventually took on Craig's book.

A very special thanks goes to my agents Yvonne Kinsella and Patricia Prizeman for seeing and believing in the message of this book and for choosing to help us get it out there. Without your help and support we don't know where this book would be. Our appreciation knows no bounds.

To Fergal Tobin for advising on and ultimately publishing Craig's book we are eternally grateful. You believed in the book, you believed in Craig, and you backed us all the way. Without you this book could be lying in a shoe box somewhere. Thank you for allowing that not to happen.

INTRODUCTION

In the inevitable and otherwise ordinary minutes that followed 2 p.m. on Monday, 26 June 2006, my life, the life of my partner and the life of our five-year-old son Craig, changed forever. It's simply impossible to convey realistically the unimaginable terror that those minutes brought. The emotion is, I believe, beyond the written word's grasp. In the turn of a breath; the beat of a heart; in the time it takes for one solitary moment to move on to the next our family was torn violently from its world of peaceful, comfortable normality and thrown upon a path of purest pain and unyielding fear that has lasted from that moment to this and will journey with us evermore.

My life up until that point was one that I can scarcely identify with now. It was blissfully normal in the accepted sense of that word; normal in its routine, in its mediocrity, in its inability to shock or surprise me in ways that were overly good or bad. My world, the life I'd built, was all about averages, predictability and the comfort inherent in such an existence. It was free from extremes. No wonderful extravagances or exuberances populated my day-to-day world nor did I expect them. Fortunes always fell at the feet of others: those unreal people who pop up in newspapers and on the television—other people. But equally misfortune was a stranger too. The horrific and unthinkable that ravaged and destroyed lives was always something I read about or heard second hand from someone who knew someone. Both of these extremes were outside the remit of my life, my world, my thinking— they had no place, they did not belong in my considerations . . . But I was wrong.

Before Monday, 26 June 2006, I had a strong personal philosophy: *It'll be grand*. I lived a life guided by my own firm conviction that no matter what difficulty came my way I'd get through it; it'll be ok. When I came into this world I was born with a *caul*. Somewhere in my upbringing I had understood this to mean that I was 'a lucky child' and so I expect this filtered down into my subconscious and forged my optimistic outlook. And so I lived my life largely with the expectation and realisation that clouds parted and sunshine followed rain . . . everything sorts itself out in the end; no sense in worrying.

Just shortly after 2 p.m. on 26 June 2006, I knew, even before I *really* knew, that something was dreadfully wrong. Barbara and I had just been told by a nurse that the consultant, whom we were expecting, was finally ready to see us. As we left Craig's hospital room several doctors accompanied us for the short walk to a more private room. And that was the moment I first encountered real fear. My stomach lurched as I sensed that this was all wrong. Not a word was said to us in those few metres between rooms . . . and so many doctors! When I looked at Barbara I knew she *knew* it too. I could see the desperation in her eyes.

When we got to the room we were told to sit down as the doctors spilled in around us, forming almost a circle. But all I could see was the doctor who was sitting right in front of me. Her expressionless face, despite itself, gave everything away. The silence of the many, the fear in Barbara's eyes, the rumbling in my stomach and the thud in my chest all ganged up on my senses and I knew that something terrible was imminent.

And then she spoke: 'Your son has a tumour in his lower brain area.' Those words affected me like nothing else in my life before. I was thrown outside myself as this terror exploded into my mind and pushed for dominance. Barbara screamed tears of utmost pain and cried out for her boy. I sat defenceless, rendered completely immobile by the gruesome reality that spread and clung deeper into my being.

And that was the beginning of a road which marked the end of all else that came before it. Everything changed from that moment on.

I'm writing these words as a man who has lost everything. Holding my son in my arms and watching his last breath slip away destroyed me. The man I am today is some reconstruction. Barbara is the same. Life after loss, after child loss, is a most gruelling, confusing and unwanted thing. It is a senseless, pointless and painful existence that is unyielding in its torment.

But love is never lost. True love never dies. It is an infinite eternal thing that transcends all and its power is beyond all that can be reasoned or conceived. There are no limitations or boundaries to contain it . . . not even death. In a world where so often we feel lost and confused, love is the only thing that is real. I've never questioned or doubted the love I have for my children.

In love, we conceived Craig. In love, we brought him into this world. In love, we shared and built our happy lives together. In love, we laughed and ran and did silly things. In love, we met our challenges together and faced them down. In love, we nursed him through his illness: through the sickness, weakness and tears. In love, he held our hands and kept shining his light and in love, we held him as he died.

But also in love, that mightiest of all things, Craig has shown us that death is not the end. In love, he has shown us that he lives on and that hope can be turned to belief. For Barbara and for me, we believe. For other grieving parents, and for everyone I suppose, I hope belief comes too.

This book is something which Barbara and I decided to do in memory of our beautiful son Craig, who left this world—who went ahead of us—on 2 November 2006.

I tried so many times before to sit down and put some words together but on each attempt I was crippled with an overwhelming sadness that forbade any clarity of thought. I guess I just wasn't ready then. But two years later I began it.

More than anything else in the world, we want this book to be a window into the life of a little boy who transformed our lives and the lives of many others who came to know him. We want the readers of this book to get a taste of the bright, thoughtful, cheeky, handsome, mischievous and witty little man who anchored such joy in our lives. His light was a bright one. We expected nothing but great things from Craig. It was always so clear to us that whatever path he would take, his personality, charisma and shining intelligence would open every door that stood in his way. But I guess he walked through one door we hadn't counted on. Craig only got to spend six years and a little over three months with us before fate took his little hand and walked him away from this world and through to another.

He was a wonderful child in life. And in death he has reached across the veil, even more wonderfully, to show us that he still lives on. He's our special Craig: an incredible, beautiful, dearly loved little boy.

This book as it is presented to you here is the very least that we, his parents, could do for him and although it is hopelessly inadequate, we've tried our best. It is but the briefest summary—notes on a life—and we can only hope that our beautiful Craig is smiling down upon it.

REMEMBERING...

Chapter 1 ~
Beginnings

I remember clearly when Craig's presence was first felt in this world. It was November 1999 and Barbara was anxious . . .

She was 'late'—in the menstrual sense of the word—and of course feared the worst. I tried to console her, endeavouring to instil my optimism that all would be fine. I, as always, couldn't possibly imagine that something as ridiculous as my becoming a father could actually happen so I never even considered the possibility. It was too ludicrous. *I'm only a child myself*, I'd thought. No, *everything would be grand.*

I tried to bend Barbara to my way of positive thinking, but she just couldn't shake off the worry. It quickly became clear to me that the only way to put an end to this growing stress was to get a pregnancy test—something Barbara didn't want to face. She was scared. I on the other hand saw it as the quick and logical solution to the dilemma: do the test, *confirm we're not* having a baby . . . happy days. It was so clean, so simple, so instant. It took me a while to actually convince Barbara but eventually we headed down to the local chemist, purchased the infamous box and set off home to put her worries to bed.

So there we were, waiting outside our bedroom for the results of the test: Barbara very concerned and me quite nonchalant. After waiting for a while we walked in together and moved over to where the test lay. *Those two blue lines;* oh how they just stared up at us—like a two-fingered gesture: silent in its delivery but menacing in its message. Our first reaction was actually nervous disbelieving giddiness. *We're going to have a baby,* we thought. Neither of us was prepared for this, nor wanted it. We laughed at it first. The enormity and significance of those two blue lines hadn't really soaked into our brains at that point. I remember we hugged each other in a 'now there's a turn up for the books' kind of way as we wallowed briefly in the short-sighted world that shock blissfully provides in such moments.

But then, later that evening, shock departed. It grabbed its things and ran for the hills. My mind, incapable just hours before of contemplating such an unfavourable outcome, was left exposed. A grim picture of life began to unfold before my mind's eye. Reality check: I was out of work, with no home and a baby on the way! Any possibilities, any career, had just been swept up and chucked into a bin. Barbara and I were to be mired within a world of constant struggle. Words like 'necessity' and phrases such as 'you've a child to provide for' all raced through my mind. The film *The Snapper* entered my head, heralding our future life, all to the depressing tune of 'Moll-eeee, my Irish moll-eee' . . . I cried.

I actually bloody cried. I cried selfishly for the optimistic future that had just been stolen. I cried for how difficult this would be for us. I hadn't cried since I was twelve but here I was utterly mortified as a 23-year-old man to be crying in front of Barbara. The situation, at this point, had turned full circle. Now Barbara consoled the blubbering *man!* in her arms, telling me, the father-to-be (those then terrifyingly unutterable words), that it would be fine. I had become momentarily overwhelmed as the pressure of life settled nicely on my shoulders, readying itself for the long journey ahead. I remember thinking I immediately had to get any old job, as long as it paid: the reality of having to sacrifice a promising life for one of toil, responsibility, bitter regret and mediocre, unimaginative survival. I *knew* that this was going to be the way. I knew this baby was coming and this unswerving reality was bearing down with every passing second.

But what I also came to realise, in time, was that I loved Barbara and she loved me and that together we would get through this. We had produced a life after all. In stark contrast to the initial despair was the slow, beautiful realisation that we had indeed created a child; that fate and circumstance had brought us together to bring about a small miracle. I'm aware that sounds completely puke-worthy but it is nonetheless true. In the following months, as Barbara's pregnancy bulged confidently forward, and the reality of the little life within became more evident, those powerful feelings were to grow even stronger.

First, however, there was the small matter of my getting a job. Within a couple of weeks I spotted something and got called. But after two rounds of interview there seemed to be an interminable wait; until finally, one morning, hope knocked on the door (rang actually). I recall with such clarity hearing the phone ringing downstairs while I was half asleep in my bed. 'Hold on, I'll just get him for you now,' my mother's voice said, as she moved up the stairs and into my room, handing me the phone. I took the call, barely containing myself as I listened to the job offer. I'd done it! I'd only bloody done it. The warmth and lightness of success folded around me and it felt wonderful. The weight of the world had just been lifted from me.

Next was the house. So in the New Year, a month or so after I'd started the job, we eagerly began looking. Neither I nor Barbara had a car (or could even drive) at that time, so with my father as driver we took a look at various properties. In the end we spotted one in Gorey which, although far from Bray, was affordable. So, monstrous mortgage now firmly clasped round our necks, we bought it.

We were so excited; a place of our own, somewhere to raise our family together. Over the following weekends we'd often ask my father for a lift down to Gorey just to walk around the outside of our new home. We had no set of keys but we didn't mind. We were thrilled just by looking in the windows and imagining how it would all be. Only a few months previously the future seemed so dismal, yet now it held such promise. This little baby, whom we didn't know, was orchestrating so many changes in our lives.

Finally there was the matter of learning to drive, and so under the guidance of my father, I began. In no time at all, and after cruising many car parks, I finally had enough confidence to bite the bullet and look for a car. We ended up buying a Toyota Yaris—which I clearly remember collecting from the garage. I recall praying there'd be no traffic (I'd never driven on a road!) but of course that would defile Murphy's Law. Instead when the window came I revved the shit out of the engine and slowly, surgically, released the clutch. The car, impressively (yet unnecessarily) loud, crawled 1 mph out onto the road and we were, well, motoring!

At this point everything was going to plan. I had a job, we had all but got our home, and after learning to drive, now had the transport sorted. All that remained was for the foetus to become a baby.

―――

Barbara had been quite sick for the first five months of the pregnancy. She had lost so much weight in that time: she'd neither an appetite nor the constitution to hold down any food. She recalls how, at about five months pregnant, she bumped into my parents in Bray as she and they were both out and about walking. My mother was immediately concerned at Barbara's appearance, asking her was she alright. She thought that Barbara looked (and to use her own words) 'malnourished and gaunt!' (It is worth pointing out at this point the vital information that my parents knew nothing about Barbara being pregnant. We had decided not to say anything until our affairs were in order.) After a chat they convinced Barbara to join them in Kennedy's pub for some food, but being relentlessly ill and never hungry she didn't have anything to eat. Not one morsel of food passed through her 'malnourished, gaunt' lips and it was then, while under the watchful gaze of my mother, Barbara feared that they were beginning to suspect something 'unusual' was afoot.

So one evening we decided it was time to goad the kitten from its bag. We were in the sitting room by ourselves, with my parents outside at the kitchen table. But isn't it strange how the mind works? I had been fine about the whole 'telling' thing, but now, at the point where the 'telling' was about to occur, I found myself unusually anxious and nervous. I looked at Barbara—who was sitting on the sofa whispering 'Go on, will ye!'—and struggled to build up the necessary courage. I couldn't believe it. Finally, in an abrupt 'this is nonsense', confident attitude, I stood up and made my way through the double doors and out into the kitchen. I looked at my parents and they looked at me. I nodded, went over to the tap, looked at it and then went back into the sitting room.

Barbara looked incredulous. 'What are you doing?' she said.

'I don't know,' was my honest reply. I laughed a little (stupidly, nervously) and then returned to the kitchen to deliver the news. But back I came again. My parents at this stage were no doubt wondering what the hell I was up to. Barbara looked fiercely at me again, her blood now pounding like thunder, and said 'Well if you don't say anything, I will!' That was enough for me. I marched straight out (again) and as my parents gazed worryingly at me, uttered the line 'We have a bit of news for you . . . we're going to have a baby.' *Done.*

Just shortly after that we told Barbara's mum and dad too. Both parents were delighted for us. We'd been worrying over nothing.

——

In late June we finally got the keys to our house and those first few weeks we spent there was a wonderful experience. The security and the freedom of having our own place, our own separate world from everyone else, was a breath of fresh air. We loved finishing work and spending the weekends there. It always felt like we were on holidays—like we'd gone away for the weekend to some holiday home. And the weather always seemed fantastic too. We were close to the beaches and the vibe in Gorey felt very holiday-ish. I'd drop down to Tesco and see people buying BBQ trays and stocking up on beer. Everyone seemed to be in shorts too and there were blue skies everywhere you looked. We loved it down in Gorey. It really did feel like a good place to call home.

On 20 July I remember sitting in the corner chair of the sitting room, scribbling away at some story I was hoping to write, while Barbara was outside in the front garden. She'd been feeling peculiar all day and had decided to do some gardening. She was sitting outside pulling up weeds and what not, and with two rosy red cheeks had the look of a grown-up (knocked up) Bosco (OHhhh Marion, Tá mé uafásach!!). I had told her to leave it but she wouldn't have it. She said she just had to do it. I remember sitting there writing away happily when I heard her calling out. I looked out the window and could see she was trying to get my attention so out I went. Turns out she couldn't get up; she was wrecked. I helped her to her feet and brought her in for a cup of tea. She was worried that she'd overdone it and was starting to feel strange aches across her stomach. Not that she was thinking they were labour pains or anything—just that she'd probably strained herself.

That night, however, at around 5 a.m. Barbara woke and told me that she was having the strange pains again. Instantly I wanted to go to the hospital but Barbara insisted she was fine and that it was probably just the effects from the gardening. So reluctantly (for me) we both turned over and tried to get some sleep, but it didn't come easy. I think about an hour and a half went by before Barbara woke up again. This time she told me that she had a 'show' and that we needed to go. Immediately we leapt into action and sped our way up the N11 bound for Holles Street Hospital.

Our 1.0L Toyota Yaris shook under the strain of the speed, I can tell you, its engine screaming as we ate up the road. I was nervous, Barbara was nervous but our total focus was on getting to the safety of the hospital. We got as far as Bray in record time and were looking good to get to the hospital in another fifteen minutes . . . until Barbara spoke.

'Just turn off here and let's go to your parents' house. I'm starving!' she said.

I looked at her with utter disbelief. 'Ye what?' is all that came out of my mouth.

'I need something to eat or I'll be sick,' she continued. 'Just do it will ye and stop arguing with me.'

Not one for arguing with a woman in labour I took the turn off, as instructed, and we ended up back in my folks' place. It was early—just after 8 a.m.—and the place was quiet. Everyone was still in bed. We found ourselves some cereal and had some tea. I kept looking at Barbara, knowing that this whole escapade was about putting off the inevitable. I could see it in her face. She was so nervous and clearly didn't want to accept that she was now going to have her baby. But with the onset of another series of pains, we hit the road again. *The pit-stop was over.*

We got into the hospital, at last, and went straight to the maternity ward where Barbara was brought for some preliminary tests and an examination. Afterwards we were brought to a room where there were two beds. There was a woman in one so Barbara took the other, as you would. A moment or so later a nurse came in and asked Barbara if she wanted anything for the pain but Barbara said she was fine. It was amazing really: within about five minutes of that moment, Barbara went—how will I put this—Ga Ga!

The pain that I witnessed was incredible. She started writhing on the bed and crying that she needed something for the torture. I ran out the door and down the corridor. I approached the nurses' station but there was nobody there. I couldn't see anybody on the corridor either. PANIC!!! *Where the fuck is everyone?* was all I could think. Just then a nurse came out from one of the wards and I ran towards her. I told her that Barbara had gone nuts with pain and that she needed something quick. She came down within a minute or so and gave Barbara some gas, which was completely useless. Barbara didn't show any signs of being relieved. On the contrary she was getting worse by the second. The nurse, however, said there was nothing further she could give.

Barbara wanted the epidural but the nurse made it clear that she simply wasn't dilated enough for that to be an option. She advised her to walk the corridors, explaining that this would help with the pain. *Bollocks* was a word I seem to remember Barbara saying about then. We did the walk though, and at one stage as we stopped for the rhythmic onslaught of pain, Barbara told me (and, in that state, I believed her!) that she was genuinely contemplating throwing herself out the window.

Another nurse told Barbara to go in for a shower and to let the hot water run on her back: this, too, would apparently help with the pain. I actually joined her in the shower room and tried rubbing her back but there was no relief to be had. It was nothing less than a sheer relentless endurance test and it was getting worse with each passing moment.

Finally Barbara was led to the delivery room. But this was by no means the end. Not by a long shot. Barbara still wasn't dilated sufficiently to permit the epidural being administered and she was to suffer hours more of this pain. She was sweating, groaning and muttering as minute by minute more and more waves of terrible pain swept over her.

At one point I recall a midwife holding Barbara's hand trying to calm her down as she made eye contact and spoke softly to her. Barbara seemed to focus on her and, on the surface anyway, seemed to benefit from this softly softly approach. So when this midwife had to move away I instinctively moved in and grabbed Barbara's hand for reassurance. For some reason, though, I didn't get quite the same reaction. In fact the image of a seventies long-haired footballer heading a ball came into my mind as I pictured Barbara leaning towards me and head-butting me right in the face. In the end though she just released her grip and threw my hand away. *Ooops!*

Eventually the anaesthetist arrived and began to administer the epidural . . . and boy did it make a difference. The transformation was extraordinary. Barbara sat up in the bed and started to speak: not moan; not wriggle or writhe; not cry. She just spoke to me. It was like she had finally emerged from some form of demonic possession—but not because *the power of Christ compelled her.* No, her saviour was that magical epidural.

A couple of hours later Barbara started to push. I was nervous at this point. I hoped to God that everything would be ok and that the baby would be perfectly formed and in full health. I remember moving to the foot of the bed and watching as the first signs of the head appeared. It was an incredible moment to be observing. I moved back up to Barbara's side as she pushed and watched as the head came slowly out. It looked like some blue elongated cone and not at all like a head, but I wasn't worried. I knew it had been contorted by its journey and would soon take shape, which it did. But it was so strange to see this little blue head just dangling out there, supported by the midwife's hands. Then, with a final push, the shoulders, followed by the entire body came sliding out. We were so happy to see that everything looked normal, and when he finally began to cry, felt a surge of relief.

It was so incredible to think that this little person was ours; that we had made him. I kissed Barbara and told her she was brilliant. She smiled and cried as she held the little boy in her arms. He was born at 7.34 p.m. and weighed in at 8 lb 6 oz. We called him Craig . . . and he was to change our lives forever.

———

It's a strange thing when first you see this little life. You don't know what you're feeling really. We certainly didn't. This little baby was ours now and we were entirely charged with his safekeeping, his happiness and his future. This little life was ours to mould and then set free. There's a new awareness that dawns on you: responsibility; and not a trivial responsibility. It's not a fleeting or passing responsibility which you can choose or discard. This is the real deal. The life and the happiness of this beautiful little soul were entrusted to us and we were entrusted with doing everything in our power to bring nothing but joy and peace to him. This beautiful little boy, our Craig, would be forever bonded to us and we to him.

Becoming a parent for the first time is perhaps the most powerful experience you can have in your lifetime. It is unlike anything else. It actually opens your eyes to life itself. You wake up from the routine of existence and are brought face to face with something greater than you. Your awareness turns away from you, your life, and begins for the first time to contemplate the eternal and the unknown. The majesty of *a* life being born into yours is exhilarating and saturates the mind with a transformed perspective on what was previously accepted and unquestioned . . . But Barbara was far too knackered to be thinking like that. She just wanted sleep.

What a day. For me, for Barbara and for our gorgeous little Craig it was nothing less than the beautiful inception to a new life of adventure and togetherness. Craig was a unique gift of perfection to our lives. His arrival into this world was a moment of undiluted elation and of deep, quiet satisfaction.

I'm a father: the thought ran over and over my mind that first night and it was a little scary too, I have to say. Like I mentioned before, I was never one for babies. I wasn't exactly drawn to them and I can say in all sincerity that I'd never ever . . . ever . . . felt broody in my life. So having one all of my own was a somewhat confusing situation to find myself in. But what I did know was that when I held him, when he opened his eyes and looked into mine, I loved him. I felt protective over him and knew that this gentle, delicate little thing looked to me and his mammy for everything he would need in order to survive in this world.

I recall how, later the next morning, a nurse came in to us with a nice warm bottle in her hand. 'Here you go, daddy!' she said, handing it to me, 'time to feed the little fella.'—my parenting was about to begin. But I must have looked stunned—I certainly felt it—as I turned awkwardly towards the cot and scuffled nervously towards Craig. I'd never fed a baby in my life. *Dear God don't drop the child,* I thought. *Don't crush his little body or choke him.* I'd never really picked up a baby before. I was anxious, to say the least, and the nurse could see it in me.

'Is this your first child?' she asked, sensing her mistake. 'Sorry,' she said, after I nodded an anxious yes, 'I just assumed it wasn't.' Now, perhaps I just had the look of someone who'd fathered many a child in his time, but I let it go! Seriously though, I was relieved to be released from the pressure.

On the Sunday we were finally let out. That first day when we got home felt lovely. It was warm and cosy and . . . easy. We were lulled, temporarily it seems, into a spirit of familial bliss and relaxed living.

We had cups of tea and relaxed in the sitting room while Craig lay sleepily in his Moses basket. It was tranquil and serene; an ambience of love and homeliness glowed about us. But when the night time came it was an entirely different matter. Pretty much from that night onwards, until Craig was about six months old, I think, Barbara and I never slept.

He was a hungry baby, you see—a savage. He was downing five bottles a night and even between feeds he made noises all night— little yelps that stunned my dead eyes into opening and fitfully surged adrenalin around my body throughout the night. I remember the big scaldy eyes on both me and Barbara as we robotically moved in and out of the bed throughout the small hours. It never ended. Night time was like a period of torture and heading to the bed was like walking to the gallows. I remember reaching a point where I genuinely considered not going to bed at all. I actually thought it would be less painful to just stay up and tend to Craig instead of enduring the endless wakeups and feeds. The constant awakenings were just killing me, but after six months it all stopped. Craig finally slept through.

——

The initial effect of becoming a father was rather a strong one for me, I have to say. I had taken a few weeks' leave when Craig was born and in those weeks I uncovered a new life. I loved being a family man. It completely transformed my view on life and how I wanted to live it. I loved spending that time with Barbara and Craig and the whole experience was just so perfect and right. All that time we had together brought us so close.

The only time I felt troubled was when I began to look to the future. I knew that the time I was spending with Craig and Barbara wasn't going to last. I knew that the happiness we shared, the beautiful closeness we felt from spending so much time together, was only some temporary illusion. In the short term I knew I would have to sacrifice this closeness and replace it with having to spend most of my days commuting the 200-km round trip to work. It began to dawn on me that returning to work in Dublin meant I would be back to early starts and late finishes. I knew that I would barely get any time with Craig at all. I'd be up and gone before he woke and would be home when he was already gone to sleep. The reality was that from Monday to Friday, and sometimes Saturdays too, my son wouldn't see me.

It killed me to think of this. Knowing that my job's location stood between me and precious time with my son, made me hate it. I resented it deeply. If I could just find something closer to home, where 9 a.m. to 5 p.m. actually meant that, I would be so much happier. But there was no changing it. There were no jobs for me in Gorey or Wexford. There were none in Wicklow either for that matter. I knew that my education and experience were only geared for Dublin and nowhere down home. I felt so trapped. Our mortgage was huge by normal standards of that time and so both of us needed to work just to keep our heads above water. This fact was the other long-term source of anguish for us both, as it meant that we'd have to put Craig into a crèche as soon as Barbara's maternity cover was finished. I can't begin to explain how much the reality of this began to hurt Barbara and me. We didn't want this.

Those first couple of weeks with Craig had felt so wonderfully simple and yet so beautifully perfect (except for the nights!). There was nothing extravagant or excessive in how we spent that time; just a new family being with each other. The taste of that experience made me long for a better life for my family. I wanted to do more than just bloody survive, chasing my time in getting stressfully to and from work—something a job in Dublin would always imply. I wanted a life of peace, purpose and fulfilment. I wanted to create a life that would offer Craig and our family so much more. I didn't want one of pointless toil and scarcity of opportunity. I didn't want Craig to grow up in the shadow of struggle and be moulded by our poor example. I wanted more than this for him, for us. But I just couldn't see how.

In truth, the birth of Craig eclipsed everything else in my life. He was my passion. It was the same for Barbara. Craig was her world. She doted over him and I'd never seen her happier. She dreaded the day that she'd have to return to work and hand him over to a perfect stranger. It would feel like the most unnatural thing in the world.

At that time crèches weren't as widespread as they are now. They were still a talking point among people and there were no real regulations governing them. The Celtic tiger had crept up on everyone in Ireland and with increasing property prices more and more parents were being forced to earn double incomes to survive. This meant a surge in crèches and I certainly couldn't escape the fear that many would be run as propitious business opportunities rather than wholesome nurturing environments for children. This was our greatest concern. We also knew of nobody else in our circle of friends or family who were using them and so we felt like such bad parents. It made us feel terrible and inadequate . . . and nervous.

But these fears and emergent regrets were unavoidable. There was no way to bypass the reality that we now lived in a very different culture to what we ourselves had grown up in. Everything in the modern world seemed faster, busier and more complex. The new life that we were about to embark on, with our beautiful little Craig, seemed fraught with great sacrifice and all for the supposed promise of a life lived in better times. Yet here, at the outset, we could only taste the former and were blinded to the latter.

———

Our new life together was many things, but a word that frequently jumps out when thinking back on that time is *struggle*. Our life was one rich in toil but poor in time; a life where we raced around from one end of the week to the next. In those earlier days when Craig was just a baby we'd be up at 5.30 a.m. I'd run out first thing and start the car, defrosting it and making sure it was warm enough before we'd head for Bray. After a long drive I'd drop Barbara and Craig off at my parents' house while I continued to the DART station. Barbara would wait until the crèche was opened and then get a lift down with my father who also dropped her up to work for her 8 a.m. start. In the evenings Barbara was finished at 4 p.m. but would have to wander around the town every day until 6 p.m., when I'd arrive back in Bray. So many hours of dead time, rain, hail or shine, every day for her. We'd collect Craig then and head off on our long drive home. We'd usually be back by 7.30 p.m., but often it was later, depending on the traffic and the many road-works going on back then.

Arriving home the routine continued: on with the dinner, eat it (while watching Craig dancing to the theme music of *Fair City*), wash and change Craig, showers, put Craig to bed, read him a story, then back downstairs to make bottles and lunches for the next day. It was just all go. It was often 10.30 p.m. by the time everything was done and by then we were just fit for bed. And in the first six months, when Craig was having his five bottles a night, this frenzy was especially hard. Barbara and I were exhausted. We were running around frantic all day and getting no sleep at night.

We battled through that every day. For the first two years I never got out once to see my friends or meet them for a drink. My life was too focused on surviving. We were broke too. All our money was spent on crèche, mortgage, petrol and other commuter costs. We had absolutely no money left over for a social life. And yet having said all that, and despite the weight of that difficult time, we remained largely content. I can say in all honesty and with perfect recollection that in spite of all the challenges, relationship tensions and hardships that certainly paved our way we grew closer as a new little family. It was difficult and stressful for sure but we always had each other.

You see, we too often take the present for granted, always racing hurriedly towards some unknown future. But had either of us known then what was lying ahead, we'd never have moved a foot. That Craig's life was to be so tragically brief was something that was hidden from us—this truth, this terrible reality lay in waiting.

Chapter 2 ❧
| Memories

Over the next six years, there were to be many twists and turns as we forged our lives together. Situations changed; fortunes altered and yet we always had each other. It was neither wonderful nor terrible . . . but it was difficult. Craig was not a perfect child and we certainly weren't perfect parents. We struggled together and did the best we could with who we were and with the situation we found ourselves in. There are regrets; too many. Barbara and I argued more than we should have, for one thing, and Craig should never have seen that. But he knew that we loved him and that we did all that we did for him. We were a family, through thick and thin, and the joys far outweighed the negative.

But I want to begin now by talking about Craig; to open that window into his life. I'm his father so I'm biased of course and there's no avoiding that. But I just want to share some of the prominent memories we have of Craig so that those who never met him can get a flavour of the boy he was and who he continues to be in that place where he has shown us he now lives on. I could talk of Craig's love of music, of singing and dancing. How he had two religions: The Simpsons and Yu-Gi-Oh. I could tell you about how emotionally intelligent, bright, caring, fair, witty, mischievous, strong and brave he was. I could just tell you this and leave it at that. But there's something Craig used to say to me whenever I tried to explain something and he got annoyed: 'Stop talking, Daddy, and show me.'

So in the next couple of chapters that is what I'm going to try and do. I am going to *show* you Craig, as best I can, through the journey we all shared through his lifetime. They are just snippets of moments in Craig's life; moments that for whatever reason have stood out in our minds and in the minds of those who knew him well . . .

Craig was always such a friendly soul. Ever since he was little he had no fear in walking up to another child and just saying 'hello'. To Craig, seeing another child was just another opportunity to get to know someone else and have some fun. It was as uncomplicated and as beautifully simple as that. There was no psychological baggage or deep-seated concern—the scars of the adult realm. His time in the crèche had taught him many things, but how to get along with others was perhaps its greatest gift to him. He was always at his happiest when surrounded by friends and family and especially other fun-loving, carefree children.

There were countless times that Barbara and I witnessed Craig approaching children and with the greatest ease getting to know them. But there is one particular memory I have that always makes me laugh, as it did so at the time. It was the time that Barbara, Craig and I visited the Dun Laoghaire Shopping Centre and Craig had his first encounter with a midget . . .

The Dun Laoghaire Midget

It was a Saturday afternoon and Craig and I were on our way to the bookshop on the first floor. We were coming out of some knick-knack shop when all of a sudden Craig began to move ahead of me. Up ahead a midget had just walked past the entrance and was walking away with his back towards us. Knowing Craig as I did, I knew that he was actually moving as fast as he was to catch up with this person to say hello. This should be interesting, I said to myself as I watched him run after the 'boy'. This midget had a generous head of curly long hair and a check shirt, so from behind he no doubt looked like a funky youngster to Craig. I watched as he ran up past the 'boy' and then stopped to turn and face him. As soon as he did I could see the whites of his eyes flaring in utter shock. His instant reaction was to run, but this time as fast he could muster and in my direction. 'PICK ME UP! . . . PICK ME UP!' he screamed as he ran and then jumped into my arms. He was crying and absolutely terrified as he looked back to where the midget was now far in the distance. He extended his arm to point in his direction and said the immortal words, 'THAT BOY HAS A MAN'S HEAD!' as he half cried in the safety of his higher perch. Well

I nearly collapsed with laughter as the honesty in his observation hit me. As I laughed, Craig's tears turned to laughter too and his grip loosened on my shirt.

I explained to Craig then that he was not a boy with a man's head, but a man like me who had just been born with shorter limbs and that he shouldn't be afraid of him. Craig understood but still wouldn't let me put him down; he didn't even want to go to the bookshop in case 'he' was there.

Over the years bedtime with Craig was always a special occasion. It was a magical time in every way imaginable and a time of great bonding for Craig and me. I loved it. Craig's room felt like a separate world, one where we both got lost in tales that were only limited by our imaginations. Yes, bedtime was story time and it was beautiful escapism for us both . . .

Bedtime Stories

In the very early years, when Craig was still a baby, Barbara would mostly be the one to bathe him and bring him to bed. At the end of a busy day it was always a nice moment for both of them to spend together. Craig loved his baths and getting into his soft cosy jam-jams. He'd smile and wriggle under his duvet, all fresh and clean and ready for sleep. As he got a little older though— pretty much from the time he could walk—I took over.

Craig would slide into bed and, as he settled into position, smile and giggle with comfort and anticipation . . . he loved that bed of his and especially that snuggling-in part. We generally had the same routine but it varied depending on whether Craig wanted a story from some book of his or if he just wanted me to make one up. Usually, before we ever got into bed there was a selection process to go through. I'd carry Craig over to his book shelf where he'd ask to see what was on offer. He'd look at the front cover, mull it over, and then ask me to pick something else. He clearly knew what he wanted; although often it felt the opposite as he rejected book after book. I'd usually speed things up at this point with a ten, nine, eight, seven countdown to no stories at all. This usually worked. Craig was a shrewd operator, you see—even at a young age—and I knew he used this 'selection time' as an opportunity to prolong the whole bedtime story period. Not that I really minded of course. I loved to watch this side of his character and see his personality flowering before my eyes.

With a book finally selected we'd get into our positions and the reading would begin. I'd sit there reading page after page, occasionally glancing and watching as his prolonged stare at the ceiling became interrupted with regular blinks. As he listened to my voice I'd watch as his big blue eyes slowly surrendered to the growing weight of tiring eyelids. I'd keep going until the long blinks stopped altogether and I knew he was finally asleep.

The problem at that point of course was getting out of the bed unheard. I'm a heavy man, there's no denying it, so any movements I made on a bed like his were always guaranteed to create a veritable fanfare of creaks and squeaks. I was about as subtle as a Siberian Yak sneaking across bubble-wrap tundra. Gauging the depth of Craig's slumber always involved running the gauntlet of this sneaky escape. Deep sleep could not be broken by my clumsy egress, but those nights were in the minority. Too often Craig was roused by the earthquake that was my un-ninja like exit from the sleepy slumberland that I'd just created. It was bordering on cruelty really: on the one hand I'd ease him into a beautiful drifting drowsiness which peacefully ended in his slack-jawed, heavy-limbed sleep; and yet just at the point where his eyes were rolling in his sockets I'd seemingly rattle the life out of the bed like some sick sleep-depriving torturer.

Many times it was impossible to know whether he was actually asleep or not. I'd stop reading, pause and look to confirm he was okay and then, just as I'd decide to make my elephantine move, I'd watch in disbelief as he'd open his eyes, look directly at me and say 'I'm not asleep. I'm just resting my eyes.' Back to square one again . . .

We read all sorts when he was younger. He had a lot of smaller books back then and it meant that I'd have to bring a few with me. He used to get bored if I just kept rereading the same one over and over so I always needed a few to interchange. I think it was because of this that I began making up my own stories for him. He loved these because they were always different and lasted longer. The interesting thing, which subsequently focused my mind, was how Craig often corrected me as I recounted different stories. He'd interrupt, saying

'No . . . that's not the way it goes,' and proceed to tell me the original storyline.

I remember the first time Craig did this and how impressed I was. I had thought that these overly long made-up stories were mostly about just hearing my voice and keeping me in the room, but having Craig correct me like that certainly changed my perception. He really had been listening and paying attention all along. It was after that I began to see just how much Craig really enjoyed these stories compared to the others.

When Craig got older these stories started to become a joint venture. Increasingly I noticed how he would often interrupt the story and tell me what he thought should happen next. He would say something like, 'No, the little boy needs to go back to the woods to find his dog first and THEN return to the shack.' And so I'd change the story. Trouble was he'd become too involved with these stories and so any notion of him being lulled to sleep was long surrendered. From the age of about three or four, the stories were no longer a tool to help him fall asleep. They were fantastic journeys, curious little tales that Craig would become so wrapped up in, his imagination, with childlike ease, taking him to some great place of adventure. I loved watching him as he listened to the stories. He was a great listener and, as I said above, a great storyteller himself. In his mind's eye he could see the story unfolding and, when required, would quietly push me in the right direction when I'd gone off track.

Occasionally, on nights when Craig was perhaps more tired than normal, we'd go back to the books and read through those. They were also the nights we tended towards more chat than story. I loved these times too; in many ways more so, in fact. We'd talk about any-thing and play all sorts of stupid and silly games. Talk would generally be about things that were on Craig's mind; questions he'd have about things he'd seen or noticed, or what someone had said to him during the day.

And the games were always fun—even though these were more of a ploy by Craig to keep me in the room. I remember making up a game that we used to play every night, last thing before I left. I came up with it as a way of maybe teaching Craig his alphabet whilst also having a bit of fun. I think he was only about four when we started it but it was a great compromise between the two of us: Craig would get to keep me in the room longer, and I'd be happy knowing he was learning his ABCs. The real truth was of course that Craig stood to gain it all.

You see I noticed that Craig had a number of posters in the room, all of which had different letters of the alphabet on them—Hulk, Spiderman, Harry Potter, Finding Nemo etc—along with some books on the bed beside us. I'd turn my back to Craig and get him to look around. Then I'd ask him to choose one of the letters he could see and to draw it out on my back with his finger. While he sketched the letter out, I was given only two guesses to get it. I'd say the letter and point to it on the wall or the book and he'd tell me if it was right or not. Over time Craig really did get to learn some of the more familiar letters and this was a real coup. But I have to say that I wasn't averse to the letters being scrawled out on my back either. I nearly fell asleep each time he did it. It was very relaxing, I must confess. At times it was I who wanted to play that game more than Craig and he was nearly kicking me out of the room.

Another game was trying to see who could come up with the most disgusting things to put on a sandwich. It always began with Imagine you were eating a sandwich and you opened it up and saw . . . ? This cropped up only every now and again but it gave Craig many laughs. Normally I'd say something like 'pooh with fingernails in it' and Craig would squirm 'Uuuugh . . .' before falling around in fits of giggles. We had so much silly fun that way, trying to top each other's choice of filling. Two kids messing around really.

Another game was 'wriggly worms'. Craig would have to put his arms over his head and I would ever so slowly approach his arm pits with my wriggling index fingers. As soon as I made contact I counted out loudly to ten, the idea being that Craig would have to last to the count of ten to be the winner. He used to collapse in hysterics when we first started doing this but before long he became an absolute master of it. There was simply nothing I could do to make him even break a smile. He'd sit there with his hands over his head as I counted to ten, only occasionally breaking the serious expression to raise his eyebrows and shoulders in a 'Is that all you've got?' expression. I on the other hand had gone the opposite way. I couldn't stand it when Craig tiggled me.

Yet another game was 'stares'. Most people are familiar with this one: two people standing opposite each other and just staring each other out until the eventual loser starts to smile or laugh. Again, Craig became a master of this. I used to flare my nostrils and try all sorts of tricks but he was like a statue. He'd beat me every single time. He was unbelievably good at it and I can't actually remember the last time I beat him.

'Head Rashers' was also an interesting concept that we enjoyed. It always began with me looking at Craig's head with a gormless expression on my face. This was always the signal that told Craig what I was up to. Before he could react I'd grab him by the shoulders and hold him still, saying 'I likes a bit of head, I do . . .' and then pull his head towards mine. I'd turn him around and just as my mouth would get to his ear I'd breathe heavily saying 'Head rashers, head rashers' and then bite into his ear cartilage (not really biting of course—that'd be just wrong!). This drove Craig mad, but he loved it. When he got older, he actually started doing this to me. I can remember the first time too. I was sitting at my computer one day while Craig was standing nearby, playing with something or other. All of a sudden I noticed he had walked up right behind me and was just standing there. When I looked at him he just looked back with a strange stare. I didn't think too much of it and turned back to whatever I was doing. But then immediately I understood. Just as the bulb had lit I heard 'Head rashers, head rashers' in my left ear. It was like a recording of someone who was whispering too close into a microphone. He also chewed my ear at the same moment. I jumped backwards, grabbing my ear and laughing as I did. Craig was in hysterics, and the seed for many such attacks was sewn.

So bedtime was always a time of fun and adventure for us both. We loved it. I think I can say that for me it was the greatest part of my day. I loved spending that time with Craig. I loved how we chatted and played and how we created so many adventures through mad stories and wild tales of all sorts. I decided at one point to record our bedtime routine. I had a minidisc player and used it to record our chats and stories. I thought it would be so good to be able to play back something so special when Craig was older. As far as I know I started these recordings when he was four. I never kept them up though and I'm so saddened by that fact. But I have over twelve hours of recordings, I think, and one day I'm sure I'll sit down to listen to them. They were precious moments and I'm glad I have them.

Invariably over the years there were times when the prospect of our long trips home to Gorey proved too much to handle. These were the tough days when our energy levels were shot and any notion of a long traffic-riddled journey ahead was just too much torment to endure. The decision to stay with my parents in Bray was usually the answer to this nightmare . . .

The Long Journey Home

Craig loved staying with his nana and granddad (or granddan as he called him). It was a bit of an adventure and a break for him from the long boring journeys each day. He was always so excited. We'd walk through that front door with Craig bellowing 'Hiya Nana,' as he walked into the kitchen. My father usually arrived in from work just after we'd all finished eating. As soon as he came in the door Craig rushed to him. 'Granddan!!' he'd shout, and run straight into him. And that was it . . . my father could never have his dinner in peace. As soon as he sat at the table Craig was over and up onto his knee. He'd sit there taking every second spoonful of his granddan's meal. He'd wriggle and squirm and my father would struggle to keep him from falling off his knee or climbing up onto the table. But granddan never complained. He loved it in fact. Despite the obvious inconvenience (and possible indigestion), he welcomed it. He wouldn't have it any other way.

So despite our frantic cries for Craig to 'stop' and 'don't be bold' he still climbed up on that knee, all perched and munching of mouth—enjoying the spoils of his victory. Once, after ignoring my instructions, he even came out with this little gem—'Yeah, but you're my daddy and granddan is *your* Daddy, so he's in charge.' The cheek of him; although I was suitably impressed with the reasoning.

But Barbara and I knew who the real culprit in all this was: Granddan. Craig always knew that he could get away with a whole lot of stuff with his granddan. As my father later said himself, he never really gave out to Craig. He didn't have the heart to. As soon as granddan was around nobody else got a look in. It was like an addiction; a two-way addiction really—they both loved each other's company.

My father remembers one night in particular when he and my mother were minding Craig while we were on a rare night out. Craig was quite young at the time, maybe two or three, and while we were out he was desperately trying to stay up as late as he could. But Nana knew better and so after giving him a nice warm bottle she brought him up to bed. She read him a story, kissed him goodnight and then left to return downstairs. Shortly afterwards—minutes perhaps—Craig tried to sneak back down but got rumbled when his Nana discovered him on the stairs.

'Get up to that bed, Craig; c'mon, be a good boy,' she said as she herded him back up the steps and into his room.

That was fine, sorted at last. A little while afterwards, maybe an hour or so, Nana decided to go up to bed herself. She was tired as she made her way quietly into her room, unaware however that little ears were listening to her every move. She closed over the door to her room and then climbed into bed. Approximately half an hour or so after she closed that door, Craig emerged from the adjacent room. He was clever enough, the little monkey, to wait out the time needed for his Nana to fall asleep. Only then did he execute his plan. Step by step he carefully and quietly made his way downstairs.

Inside in the sitting room my father was completely unaware of what was going on. This was at least an hour and a half, or more, after Craig had been put to bed. My father was sitting on the sofa looking at the TV in the corner of the room, when through the frosted glass doors that led into the kitchen he could see the unmistakable silhouette of a cunning little boy. I don't believe it! he thought as the doors then slightly opened to reveal Craig's face.

'Sshh,' Craig said instantly, with his finger up to his dody-filled mouth. 'Nana is in bed,' he continued, completely unconcerned as to whether or not his granddan might put him to bed too. He obviously knew better.

He then calmly walked over, snuggled in beside his granddan on the couch and stayed up until the wee hours. The expression 'thick as thieves' was coined for these two. Actually, in the mornings Craig would often go into his granddan too. He'd climb into the bed beside him and through the walls we could hear him yapping away. They were inseparable, they really were.

When Craig was a little older, staying in Bray sometimes had other benefits. I'm thinking in particular of the few times when Barbara had a work function in Bray to go to. Usually Barbara and her friend, Gillian, would go out together on those nights and then come back to sleep in the sitting room in my parents' house. Gill fondly recalls how generous and charming Craig was to her. When she and Barbara were finally all dressed up and ready to go, Craig—without fail—would always say, 'Mammy you look lovely,' and 'Gillian you look so nice.'

I'd usually drop them down to the pub, first stopping off to collect another friend, Olwyn, on the way. Craig of course would be in amongst all the women in the back seat loving the attention and the atmosphere. I remember the first time I brought Craig with me in the car when dropping the girls down. He was all giddy and excited to begin with but quickly felt rejected and sad when they spilled out of the car and left him. He'd assumed he was going with them and was disgusted with them.

There was another time like this I can recall where Craig really tried it on. He had a Muscle-Spiderman outfit that he'd gotten for Hallow-een and which he'd often wear every now and again just for fun. Anyway on this particular occasion he brought it with him to Bray knowing that we were going to be staying the night. Barbara and Gillian were going to a fancy dress party that night, as it happened, and they had their outfits ready to go. Barbara was dressing up as some kind of burlesque lady and Gillian as a naughty nurse. When Craig saw them in their outfits he immediately rushed to get his Spiderman outfit. On the way down in the car to drop the girls off Craig began pleading with them to bring him into the party too. 'Look, I'm dressed up and everything,' he begged. Barbara felt sorry for him but told him he wouldn't be allowed into the pub, that children couldn't come in that late at night.

'But they won't know I'm a child,' he said, 'not with this mask.'

But it wasn't to happen. Barbara explained it wasn't up to her—it was the law. Craig was so angry. He sat there in silence for about a minute, only breaking it to say 'Yeah well, when I get older I was going to bring you out with me, even though you would be really really old. I wouldn't have cared . . . but now I'm not!' he exclaimed, before folding his arms in utter disgust.

However, just knowing that Gillian was staying the night was usually enough to keep him happy. He always had a plan of action for this too. The sleeping arrangements on those nights were always the same: Craig and I would be upstairs sharing the same room, with Craig in the top bunk and me in either the bottom bunk or the single bed. Barbara and Gillian would sleep downstairs in the sitting room. My mother would leave out sheets, pillows and a duvet and I would always make up a bed on the floor for them before going to bed myself. I'd usually keep my phone on and wait for the 'Can you give us a lift up?' call that usually came at about 2 a.m. and then pop down, in my pyjamas, and get them.

But this wasn't the only night activity that went on during those nights. While lying asleep in my bed I'd always be gently awoken by the stealthy movements of one Craig Sexton as he climbed down the ladder. If I was on the bottom bunk I'd open an eye just in time to see two little feet appear on the top rung near my head. I'd watch as they moved with great care, searching out each lower rung with deliberate subtlety before committing to the required pressure for a silent descent. I'd watch with one eye open, seeing Craig reach the floor and pausing to look in at me.

'What are you doing?' I'd mumble.

'Going down to Mammy and Gillian,' he'd say, before making his way to the door and continuing downstairs.

This was usually six in the morning or so. He did this every time Gillian stayed over. Some nights I'd only be woken by the noise of the door-handle being pulled en route downstairs. I'd smile knowingly and then close that eye again.

Downstairs Craig would quietly open the sitting room door and clamber through the darkness and over the duvet before finally squeezing in between the two sleeping women. Barbara would often put the TV on for him and he'd happily stay there until they were ready to get up. He just wanted to be a part of the gang I suppose and loved snuggling in with them. It's no secret either that Craig wasn't averse to having Gillian's boobs close by. I believe he was very much the fan. He'd always been an admirer of the female boob actually. I guess he just liked the feel of it. In fact before going asleep Barbara would always remark to Gill that Craig would be coming down for a 'squeeze' in the morning.

In fact there was one occasion where Gillian was having a shower in the house in Bray. Craig, standing outside the bathroom, decided that he was going to walk in. 'You can't go in there, Craig. Gillian's having a shower!' Barbara said, pointing him away from the door.

'But I just want to have a peek at Gillian's boobies, that's all,' he said, as innocent and honest as you like.

But Gill thought the world of Craig. She knew he was just a beautiful, funny and charismatic little boy who for her was such a joy to be around.

When Craig was about three years of age he was an energetic little fella. Like most three-year-olds he was full of adventure and wonder and so his little legs would often carry him to places that were not exactly, well . . . safe! Plus the beauty of being that age is the wonderful clarity of thought that guides your decisions—if you want something, you go after it; if you're not happy with something, you let it be known and if you're eager to go some place, well off you go. Decisions are simple, not complex, and the term *consequence* has no meaning whatsoever. Black or white; yes or no; stay or go. I can think of no better example of this wonderful attribute than the time Barbara took Craig for a walk up the town in Gorey.

Run Forrest Run!

It was a Friday and Fridays always meant mammy and Craig time in those early years. Craig, as always, was looking forward to spending the day at home and getting a chance to be outside in the fresh air— something of a rarity when in the crèche.

On this particular day they both set off as normal on their walk up into the town. They'd usually have a look around the shops and then go for 'something nice' in Joanne's—for Craig this nearly always took the form of a particular bun with a deliciously soft caramel icing on top; oh how he loved that bun. So off they went out of the house, down through the estate, across the busy Coach Road and up through Esmonde Street. They walked along, chatting their usual chatter as they went, and happy in each other's company. But just as things unfolded as they ought to, Craig decided to change the status quo.

With not the slightest inkling as to what was about to happen next and with absolutely no reason for doing so, Craig turned around.

'I don't want to go up the town,' he said.

'Why not?' Barbara asked, surprised by this. 'Do you not want to go for a cup of tea and a cake?'

'No,' and with that he ran.

'Craig!' Barbara called, shocked to see him running off, 'get back here now!'

But it was incredible. He just kept running. Barbara hadn't anticipated this. She thought he'd run a little bit, then stop, but no. He just took off. Barbara then took to running after him, shouting after him in her pursuit, but the little man just kept going. Barbara, a former All-Ireland medallist for running, just couldn't catch him. His pace was constant and unrelenting. Barbara's heart was in her mouth as he ran off into the distance and towards the busy road and roundabout. She was terrified and yet there was nothing she could do. She watched as he moved further towards that busy road, apparently homeward bound, but very much into the jaws of danger. He just kept running and running. The only time he stopped was when he reached the road.

Barbara could see him in the distance. At least he had had the good sense to check the traffic before crossing. He crossed that road! Barbara thought, her fear now turned to anger as he continued his run safely into the estate. She was fit to kill him of course by this point. He had been so unbelievably bold and so careless.

Eventually she made her way up through the estate and finally turned into the driveway of our house. There he was. Sitting on the front step he looked up and said only two words, 'I'm sorry!'

Oh he knew he was in trouble all right. Barbara took him into the house and gave him an extremely thorough lecture on just how spectacularly bold he had been. 'Why did you run off like that?' Barbara asked, but all Craig could say was 'I don't know . . . I just didn't want to go up the town.'

When enough 'punishment' time had passed—enough for the message to sink in, that is—they did actually go up the town and had a very pleasant time as it turned out.

In the summer of 2003 we decided that we were taking Craig on his first foreign sun holiday—Menorca. I wasn't too hot about going on any sun holiday if the truth be told. Nature blessed me with the type of skin suited only to caves and shadows and so the idea of basking in the sun was abhorrent to me. Barbara, on the other hand, is a sun worshipper. She could lie out in the sun all day and be perfectly content. While Barbara spent her time relaxing under the sun, I spent mine trying to fight it off. Smothered in creams, like some basted chicken, I'd curse the menacing blob of lava overhead that promised only stroke and cancer . . . and pain!

The Menorca Moment

So anyway, off we headed to the sun, Barbara and Craig positively bursting with excitement and anticipation. We were a little anxious that the long plane journey would prove too rigid and containing, causing Craig to explode into some screaming, spitting and fitting devil child at 20,000 metres. Quite why we envisaged that particular level of discord I don't know, but perhaps the collective consciousness was whispering to us that the combination of two-year-old boy, confinement and over two hours of travelling was a particularly horrific alchemy. As it turned out, though, our concern was over-whelmingly misplaced. Craig was the very model of best behaviour.

That first hurdle being overcome set a nice tone for the holiday. Even I was feeling less apprehensive—despite Lucifer's unclenched orifice of a sun excreting its constant hellish load from the sky above. Barbara was smiling away, content that she was here in the Mediterranean and that a week of sun lay ahead. Craig was just excited.

After settling into our room we came back out and got two beds by the pool. Like I said it was really busy and every corner of the pool side was occupied. Sitting on the edge of the bed Barbara started putting cream all over Craig. As she did so Craig's eyes were fixed on the kids' pool on the other side. There were kids jumping in and out of the water, laughing and playing and having a lot of fun. The beds we had were located right beside the deep end of the pool and, knowing that Craig couldn't swim, this was far from ideal. We knew we'd have to watch him like a hawk. It was a long enough walk around to the kids' pool on the other side and there was no way we could let him go there on his own. Barbara couldn't swim either so I knew it was up to me.

Just as I was in the middle of getting my bed ready and putting on cream I heard Barbara saying 'Craig come here!' I turned around and could see that Craig had walked away from Barbara.

'Craig, get back here!' I said forcefully, as he had begun to move forward even more. He was still looking at the other kids who were in the water swimming and playing. It was like he was mesmerized.

'Craig!!' Barbara said loudly, panic in her voice as he just moved further towards the edge of the pool.

Then the unspeakable happened. It was almost in slow motion. Craig moved to the edge of the pool, leapt into the air and went under the water.

'CRRAAAIiiigggg!' Barbara screamed, as I ran towards the pool. 'JESUS, NEVILLE, GET HIM!'

I grabbed Barbara by the arm and made sure she didn't jump in. The last thing I wanted was her drowning us all. I didn't want to jump in on top of Craig either so I jumped to the left of the bubbles which fizzed in Craig's wake and made sure I didn't go all the way down. Once in the water I dipped my head under and looked down to see where he was. I could see him at the bottom looking up at me with his blue eyes. I lunged downwards and reached under his armpits, pulling him up. When he got to the surface he let out an enormous roar and he pulled tight into my neck.

'I couldn't breathe,' he said, between tears and panic. 'I thought I was going to die,' he whimpered.

He kept crying as I lifted him out of the pool to his mammy who took him and hugged him desperately. I could see there was a man standing at the edge of the pool too. He was ready to jump in to assist if necessary by the looks of it. After I climbed out I moved to the beds and tried to calm down. I couldn't believe what had just happened. My heart was racing with the thoughts of what could have been.

'What did you do that for, Craig?' we quizzed, as he began to calm down.

'I just saw everyone else doing it so I did it,' he said. 'I didn't know it was going to be like that.'

'You have to learn how to swim first,' we told him. 'You could have died, darling. Promise you won't ever do that again, you hear?'

'I promise,' he answered, as he snuggled in beside his mammy and lay out on the bed with her. He had clearly been frightened by the experience and just wanted to be comforted. Barbara and I felt the same, I can tell you. We could have done with some hugs and comfort too. We were in shock. That one incident actually tainted the rest of the holiday for us. I was on high alert the whole time we were there.

I couldn't believe it then when only after about twenty minutes Craig got up from his mammy's side and said that he wanted to go up to get in to the kids' pool. I was amazed. In one way I was relieved: relieved that he hadn't been scarred by the incident and was apparently not in any way terrified of the water. This was a good thing. The other part of me was just concerned. We both were. We were afraid that he would put himself in a dangerous situation again.

I walked him up to the pool and watched as he climbed straight in. The pool was deep enough to be dangerous to a non-swimmer, that was for sure. I knew Craig could easily lose his balance and wouldn't be able to right himself so I had to sit with him, ever vigilant, as he paddled about with the other kids. As I sat there on the edge I was actually amazed at the resilience he'd shown. All he wanted to do was play with the other kids. This was his driving force. This is what moved him to action. He was in that pool so that he could play with the other kids, not for the water itself. I had to admire his grit and determination.

The night that Craig woke up crying and telling us that he had a ghost in his room proved to be a very interesting and memorable night indeed. It was back in the spring of 2003 and it was a typical Friday night . . . or so we thought . . .

The Ghostly Visitor

We had put Craig to bed at his normal time and after watching some trashy Friday night TV we headed up to bed ourselves. All was fine, normal I guess, and in no time at all we were both fast asleep. I think it was several hours later when we were woken by a startling noise. It was Craig. He was crying in his room and so Barbara leapt out of the bed and ran into him. Craig would sometimes have nightmares and so this wasn't entirely unfamiliar territory for us. Barbara stayed with him in the room until he fell asleep again and then returned to our bed.

'He said he'd seen a man standing in his room, looking down at him—a ghost!' Barbara told me as she climbed under the duvet. 'I told him he was just having a nightmare and waited until he drifted off. He's fine now—fast asleep.'

I turned over, reassured, and tried to get back to sleep. I was wrecked tired and knew I had a Saturday shift to cover in the morning so just wanted to go back to sleep. I must have drifted off fairly soon after this, but it wasn't long, an hour or so perhaps, before I heard Craig crying again. I went straight into the room and after sitting with him for a little bit figured he needed a drink, so I headed downstairs to get him a bottle. When I got down there I couldn't believe what I was looking at. The kitchen counter was littered with mini Kia-Ora orange cartons. Most of them were still within the plastic wrapping but two or three were thrown across the counter top. My initial thought was that Barbara must have come down earlier while I was asleep to get one of those drinks. It was so uncharacteristic though for Barbara to leave them out like that and in such a heap. I was half asleep and didn't really dwell on it, to be honest. Just then I walked out into the utility room to get to the fridge. When I entered the room I just couldn't believe what I saw. The fridge door was wide open—for how long I'd no idea. Jesus, Barbara must have been in some state to leave everything like this, I said to myself. I couldn't understand how she would have done this. She'd never do anything like that and it baffled me. Before heading back upstairs I cleaned away the juices and closed the fridge door, shaking my head in disbelief. When I got back upstairs and finished with Craig I jumped back into bed. I said something to Barbara and heard her mumble something in return about not having a clue what I was talking about. Anyway, I was too tired and just went back to sleep.

Again, however, sleep wasn't for long. I woke up after hearing a noise. Barbara heard it too. We could hear footsteps out on the landing. Straight away I knew Craig was out of his bed and on his way to climb into the bed with us. He often did this, coming over to my side of the bed and rolling over my shoulder to snuggle in between us. But as we lay there, there was no sign of Craig coming in. And still we could hear the noise of footsteps outside in the landing. Barbara and I looked at each other with a kind of What's he up to out there? expression on our faces. But then the noise stopped. What followed sent a chill down my spine. As we lay there the distinctive sound of a man going for a piss rang in our ears. What the fuck? I thought. Craig was not yet three and he could only sit on the toilet when he needed to go. This was a man going to the toilet in our house. I raced out of the bed, with Barbara crying behind me incapable of believing her ears. I went out to the landing and looked into the bathroom. The light was on and there, with his back to me, was a strange man standing over the toilet.

'Ehh . . . Hello,' I said, as I walked into the bathroom behind him. Immediately though I became paranoid that this was some ploy just to lure me into the toilet while this man's accomplice readied himself to club the back of my neck. So as soon as that thought reared its head I ducked and turned back to look behind me. But the coast was clear. It was comical really. Back in our bedroom I could hear Barbara saying 'Oh JESUS!! . . . I'm ringing the Guards,' and could hear her making her way past me to go downstairs.

'Stay where you are!' I said to Barbara. I didn't want her going downstairs—just in case—but also knew that we didn't need to ring the Guards at all. I could smell the stench of alcohol off this guy and when he had turned to face me I could see that his eyes were bloodshot and unfocused. I knew he was no burglar, just some drunken fool who had wandered into the wrong house. I knew my neighbour had a lodger, so seeing this man before me I was certain this was him; he had obviously drunkenly wandered into our house. Quite how he got in I wasn't sure but for me the danger was over. I questioned him but he was barely able to speak. All he could mutter was my neighbour's name and that was enough for me. I brought him downstairs and put him out the door, smiling to myself.

Everything about that night started to add up then. The open fridge; the scattered juices; Craig saying there was someone in his room. This guy was responsible for all of it. Not long after I let this fella out I had to get up for work but later on that day Barbara rang me to tell me that the guy had been into our back room too and that he'd pissed all over a clean basket of clothes. She was furious and I couldn't blame her.

But in a curious twist of fortune I actually won €320 on the Grand National that day. A memorable day indeed and Craig got his cut of it too—he managed to drill home the fact that we hadn't believed him about the man in his room and so some form of compensation was warranted!

Chapter 3

Moments

On 2005 we decided that we were going on another sun holiday. Our trip to Menorca back in 2003 had been a somewhat mixed bag for Barbara and me but there was no doubt that Craig had loved it. So, it was with this in mind that we decided to go back to the sunnier climes that year.

Sun, Sun, Sun . . . Here We Come

Ordinarily the idea of a package sun holiday is something that makes me cringe. On every level it is the perfect anti-holiday for me: beautiful hot days (I hate the heat), basking in the sun (my skin is useless. If I dream of the sun I wake with sunstroke) and relaxing by the pool or beach (can't really relax or read—it's too bloody hot!). I just wasn't designed for sun holidays and it's as simple as that.

This time, however, after our experience with Craig in Menorca, I was super anxious about the whole thing. The last trip had felt like I was on permanent lifeguard duty—watching Craig's every move as he walked and ran within a metre of the edge of the pool. I remember I'd brought three books with me to read, and only reading about twenty pages in total. Barbara would lie out, lizard-like, getting browner by the second and I'd hide under the parasol with my eyes constantly on Craig. As Barbara couldn't swim it was down to me to be supremely vigilant. I think it's telling that when we finally had to leave Menorca I actually found myself excited, looking forward to getting back—how unbelievably sad is that. That's a real measure of that holiday.

So I knew Lanzarote, where we finally decided upon, was going to be more of the same. But, that being the case, I put my own complete lack of excitement aside and was happy enough, knowing that Craig would enjoy himself. He deserved the break away. As long as we were all together, no matter where it was, what did it matter! Craig had been anticipating the holiday ever since he knew it was booked. Conversations were always littered with 'How many more weeks until our holiday?' and 'How long will we be there for again?' as he tried to feed his enthusiasm. It was great to see actually—I only wished I'd felt the same.

When we got to Lanzarote the sun was in full flight. Barbara was beaming and Craig was reeling with anticipation. I was, well, *there*, let's say. No more, no less. Although actually that's not entirely true either. I was looking forward to something different. I suppose just to get away from the normal rigours of our life was very welcome, so in actuality I was in good form.

Our room was pleasant enough and we were right beside the pool so our first impressions were pretty good. It seemed cosy and relaxed and within easy reach of everything. The first thing we did after settling in was to get out and about to get a feel for where we were. We weren't too far from the beachfront either, just a few minutes' walk. As we made our way there, moving through the streets and roadways, I was struck by the intensity of the heat. Craig felt it too. I can still see his face as he looked up at the sky and said those unforgettable words—'That sun is as big as the earth'—while pulling at the collar of his t-shirt. Barbara and I just laughed.

Craig was blessed with a lot of my pigmentation and so his heat tolerance (intolerance) was similar to mine. But boy what a difference a hundred metres made. As we turned onto the promenade there was an immediate gush of cooler air. It swept up along the entire beachfront and, coming in off the ocean, was almost vapour-like. It was beautiful. I could have stayed out all day with a wind like that. Craig was the same. 'Oh that's lovely, isn't it,' he said, his head tilting skyward allowing the wind to cool the heat beneath his chin. This was actually a defining moment for me. It set the mood for the entire trip as with that life-giving breeze there came a most pleasant realisation—this is going to be good!

We continued down to the beach and walked out onto the sand. It was boiling hot but the sea breeze was even more generous down there. In Menorca there had been no beach; just that pool. I had forgotten how different sitting by the pool and lying out on the beach were from each other. As we strolled along cooling our feet in the lapping water and feeling the rush of wind on our faces we felt refreshed. There was none of that dead heat that one endures by the pool; just an easy pleasant comfort. It was the first time I understood the phrase *a relaxing holiday in the sun*.

That week was to become the best sun holiday that I ever had. As a family holiday it really couldn't have been any better. Barbara and I have so many wonderful memories of that time together. Such happiness, such joy and all because of how much Craig got out of it. He was without doubt the star of that trip.

He couldn't have enjoyed himself anymore if he tried. He loved the fact that he was able to go out with us at night. This for him was the best thing in the world ever. All those nights where Barbara would go out with Gill and Olwyn and not bring him; those nights where I'd be out and he'd be stuck at home; every single one of those nights had built up to this holiday, and boy did he let loose! Craig would have been only four, maybe five, when we were in Lanzarote, but that was in no way a restriction for him. In fact he was out with us every night until 3 a.m.

The evenings always began the same. We'd find a nice restaurant along the beach front where we'd settle in for a nice meal and some banter. A warm wind blew each evening, carrying on through the night as we ate and providing the perfect balance of temperature. After the meal it was time to hit the bars. The fantastic thing about Lanzarote is that it is so child friendly. Most, if not all of the bars and clubs were littered with other families so there was an easy relaxed vibe as we moved from one to the next. Craig would sit there, like the giddyboots he was, smiling and looking all around him. He was so wonderfully ecstatic just to be out and about where all the adults were.

But it was never long before Craig was up on his feet and moving to the music. He loved dancing. It was in his blood. Ever since he was an infant in his walker dancing to the theme tune to *Fair City*, we knew music was in his bones.

In each bar we went to the music blared out from the speakers and Craig was powerless to resist. He'd just have to get up. His body wouldn't allow him to sit still. We were mesmerised by his energy and his determination to dance and he was never shy about it either. He'd just march up to the dance floor and get his grove on.

There was this one particular bar that we went into which had a central dance floor made completely out of chequered tiles of constantly changing lights. The tiles would change colour and often to the rhythm of the music being played. When Craig got inside he was in his element. He was actually the one who dragged us in. When we'd first walked in to the bar the dance floor was empty. Lots of people, including other kids, were sitting in the relative din surrounding the colourful mosaic. Nobody was brave enough, it seemed, to get up. Craig watched from his seat, falling deep into thought as we sat there with our drinks. He looked around him and then noticed that not only was there this magnificent dance floor, but also raised podiums on the corners of it each topped with a single large lit tile. Like the dance floor below them these podium tiles changed colour. It proved irresistible. He got up out of his seat, climbed up onto the podium, and began his dance.

People looked at him from around the room but he didn't give a damn. He just looked over at us, a nervous but determined smile on his face, and kept busting his moves. It was funny actually. Just before he got up he asked his mammy to roll up one of the legs of his ¾ length shorts. He had a temporary tattoo on the calf of that leg and wanted to show it off while he danced. We sat laughing, watching as he kept that leg to the front so everyone could see his 'cool' spider tattoo.

Probably the greatest compliment Craig received was the night we went to an underground nightclub and he almost danced himself into a coma. The club was extremely family friendly with lots of kids running around the place, but also with a good balance of regular party goers. There was a great atmosphere and Craig, as always, was bursting with enthusiasm as we found our seat. This particular night there was a DJ up on the stage playing a good variety of music while on the other side of the room they had an inhouse dancer gyrating and kicking over on a raised platform. The night was primed for enjoyment.

After ordering our drinks and taking maybe one or two sips, Craig's hand (as always!) grabbed his mammy's and began pulling her towards the dance floor. He was chomping at the bit and had enough of the sitting around nonsense. He wanted his hooves on that floor and that was that. Unfortunately, however, Barbara was far too sober at that stage to get up and dance in front of a massive audience, so she had to decline. But Craig was insistent. Unlike him, however, Barbara needed to consume a hell of a lot more chemical confidence before starting that lark. Ever determined, and not one for giving up, Craig was relentless. Surrounded by other tables—all of which were packed with people now watching Barbara being pulled by the hand—Craig deliberately spoke louder and pulled with all his might as he 'begged' her to get up with him. The scene was set. Craig had made it impossible for her to say no and so reluctantly, and with the empty laugh of one on the brink of humiliation, she allowed herself to be dragged to the floor.

I looked out from the comfort of my seat and thanked the gods that it was her and not me. As soon as the song was finished Barbara made her move to leave. However, that didn't quite fit in with Craig's plans so she stayed. Deep into this second song Barbara began to thaw out. Limbs and muscles, only moments before rigid with mortification, began to melt into the music and the atmosphere. With complete abandonment Barbara let loose and tore up the dance floor with Craig. She flung him around; twisting and turning him this way and that as his body flailed and flapped in response. He was ecstatic. I could actually hear his laughter through the music from where I was sitting. Everyone else watching on could hear it too. Craig was being flung around like a rag doll, delirious with the joy that filled his heart. He was so happy.

They both stayed up on that floor for ages. More people began to fill it then and it was only out of exhaustion that Barbara returned to her seat. Craig came back too, but took a few sips of his drink and then went straight back up by himself. At this stage he was a force unleashed. Above the dance floor, just in front of the DJ box, he and a few other kids began to dance on the stage. They were hyper, throwing themselves around and jumping up and down. Eventually the inhouse dancer came down to the stage and, leading Craig and the kids behind him, with the adults to the front, began a dance routine.

As the song played and the dancer led, Craig followed his every twist and turn. He was brilliant. He did it so well that the DJ actually spoke over the music to single him out and say how impressed he was. Craig's reaction was priceless. He looked down to us, sitting in our seats, and smiled the cheesiest smile of satisfaction. We stood up, gave him the thumbs up and cheered him on (we'd had a few beers by then!).

A little later on that night all the kids were asked back up onto the stage by the DJ. They were to be the entertainment for everyone watching on as they danced to the different tunes that the DJ played. For a laugh the DJ occasionally announced that he wanted them to dance a certain way: fast, slow etc. while he played the relevant music. This was a great source of amusement for everyone watching on and we all laughed and cheered as they did it. But it was only when he played a really slow sexy song that Craig had everyone glued to him. While all the other kids kept leaping and jumping like rain splattering on a path, Craig slowly ground his hips in a circle and wriggled his entire body. It was both compelling and hilarious. The DJ couldn't get over it. He spoke into the microphone saying, 'Look at this kid; what a mover!' and pointed from his booth to Craig whose hands were now behind his head as he gyrated and pursed his lips to the music. The DJ looked to the podium where the inhouse dancer was doing his thing and again announced over the microphone, 'Carlos, I think we've found your replacement. You better watch your back. What a mover eh?'

Barbara and I couldn't have been more proud. Craig loved it all. All night he dragged his mammy up and down to that dance floor; he just didn't want to stop. At one point he came back to the table to get a drink. He stood, leaning against his mammy, still looking out onto the floor whilst taking a well overdue breather. As Barbara and I were talking I happened to look at Craig and could see that he was closing his eyes. Like a horse, he was starting to sleep standing up. I nodded to Barbara to look at him and as soon as she saw him with his head falling forward and eyes shut she said, 'C'mon, time to go home. You're knackered,' and pulled him into her. But with that Craig sprang back into life.

'No, not yet,' he said, fighting off the heavy slumber and moving straight back out on to the dance floor.

'The little divil,' Barbara said, turning to me. 'He just doesn't know when to stop, does he?'

Craig stayed up there on that floor for another half an hour, I'd say, before coming back for a drink. This time he sat in his chair and it wasn't too long before we could see his head getting too heavy for his neck. *It was time to go!*

It was just after 3 a.m. and he was shattered. He had literally danced himself to a standstill and had nothing left to give. I had to carry him in my arms and was dreading the long walk home. Craig was a hardy chap and it was a long walk; thankfully though we managed to get a taxi.

But, tired as he was, Craig was still as sharp as a tack. Inside the taxi he sat at one door and I at the other, with Barbara in the middle. When we got to our stop I opened my door and we all climbed out on my side. Craig was furious with us.

'Why did you do that?' he quizzed, Barbara and I not knowing what he was talking about. 'I was the last one out of that back seat and that man could have driven off with me, when you two were out. Next time I'm sitting in the middle, so I can get out whichever side first . . . Ok?'

It was just another example of how observant and deep thinking Craig could be. He never ceased to amaze us in that respect.

We returned to that club a few times that week—chiefly because Craig fancied the promotion girl outside it who, incidentally, gave him a kiss each night he was there—but visited many more besides.

Our days that week were spent at the beach where Barbara sunbathed and Craig and I hid under the parasol. It was funny really. Every day a local Spanish guy would walk up and down the stretch of beach trying to sell ice-creams to the huddled masses. And every day as he approached where I lay he would shout out—with everyone listening—'Ehh . . . big white chickennnn . . . eh!' It was funny the first time, even amusing the second time, but from then onwards I wanted to kill that man. Craig would laugh and warn me: 'Here he comes, Daddy!' and then smile at his mammy as he waited eagerly for the 'show' to begin. So that was part of the everyday too, and although I frequently had murder on my mind as a result, it never took away from the enjoyment—much.

Craig and I spent a lot of time in the water ducking and jumping under waves. He'd grab me by the neck and we'd wait for a big one. As soon as it came we'd drop and let it crash over our heads. It was such a laugh and Craig loved it. If he'd had his way, we'd never have left the water at all.

It had been a beautiful holiday in every way possible and when we left we promised to return again. Sadly, that was never to be.

As I've mentioned already, with our lives so choked up with work, crèche and commuting our small bit of family time was very limited indeed. Routine became the cornerstone of everything we did. From the moment we woke up in the morning to when we finally fell into bed at night we followed a clockwork operation. Part of this daily routine was Craig's shower, which always came shortly after dinner. I have so many wonderful and humorous memories about those showers that I think it only right to share some here.

Shower stories

The first thing to explain is that pretty much from the moment Craig could walk he had a shower every day—and with me! We'd go upstairs, turn the shower on and the race would start. The competition was to see who could get undressed first and jump into the shower. We did this every single time and I grew to learn over time that Craig absolutely hated losing. He simply did not like it one bit. As a result, and to avoid a thunderous mood, I mostly let him win. I'd pretend to get stuck inside my shirt or go so deliberately slow that Craig always just about eked in front of me. He'd stand there naked— hand on hips (like a superhero) for a moment—then run to the shower where he'd laugh with greedy triumph.

Occasionally though I'd mix it up a little, just to keep things interesting, you understand. Normally the race would begin with a nod or a knowing stare that implied it was 'on'. But sometimes after turning the shower on, and with no notice whatsoever, I'd just shout 'GO' and then begin to rip every shred of clothes off me, leaving Craig for dust. He'd stand there, saying 'NO!' at me as I furiously removed garment after garment. 'No . . . that's not fair, Daddy, . . . I'm not playing . . . that doesn't count,' he'd whine, but all the while he was growing more and more angry as he watched me ignore his pleas and continue to pull off all my clothes. He'd be seething, disgusted with me for this deliberate and calculated manoeuvre and I'd watch the fury burning in his eyes as he stood there with arms folded, resolutely boycotting the competition. I'd remove almost every stitch in lightning time, but then stop when I'd get to my socks. I'd pretend to get stuck with them. I'd watch then as Craig's look would start to soften, with the temptation to start undressing clearly crossing his mind. I'd continue to fumble with the socks and hop on one leg outside into the landing. I'd even swear as if to highlight how annoyed and frustrated I was becoming. I'd glance back into the room and smile quietly to myself at the scene before me: Craig tearing his clothes off.

I'd shout in at him, 'Hey hold on, we're not playing anymore . . . you said you weren't playing!' and watch as he just laughed with such excitement and nervousness as he tried with monumental effort to snap victory from the jaws of hitherto certain defeat. I'd laugh to myself as I witnessed the sheer concentration of will and the fervent anticipation of victory in his every move. It was like a person being fast forwarded. I'd wait until he'd get to his socks and then I'd run into the room and pull him onto the bed, trying to hold him down. I'd hold him with one arm and let him watch as I managed to remove one of my socks. This raised the stakes and although Craig would be angry with me for 'cheating' like this, he would be in fits of giggles. Then I'd purposely let him slip from my grasp and watch his bubbling elation as he'd break away, rip off the socks and then pose with hands on hips and bottom lip over top. The last thing I'd see was his little arse disappearing into the shower to claim his victory.

The shower itself of course was another source of great fun. I can remember a couple of incidents in particular which are worthy of a mention here. Craig would always stand in the left hand corner of the shower tray while we had our showers and most of the time he'd be singing or talking away to me about different things. I'd normally wash myself first, letting Craig just stand under the warm water and relax for a while, and then afterwards I'd wash him. On one occasion, however, I remember standing there washing myself, lost in thought about something or other, when I suddenly became aware of a silence. This was not normal. I looked down through the suds and could just about see Craig's blue eyes facing towards and up to me. He was smiling at me and I was confused. 'What?' I said. But as soon as I said it my peripheral vision took in the golden stream that was arced across my knee. The little rascal was peeing on me! 'You little monkey!' I said and moved my leg away while Craig burst into fits of laughter. He laughed so hard that he nearly slipped in fact. It didn't bother me of course, not in the shower anyway. However, when I turned to Craig and showed him what was dangling not far from his head, saying 'That was a silly thing to do now, wasn't it!' Craig's expression changed in an instant.

'No Daddy, don't . . . I didn't mean it,' he pleaded but laughing as he turned away from the loaded gun that was pointing menacingly in his direction.

Actually on that topic I must mention a peculiarity of Craig's. It was a funny thing actually. He'd occasionally share showers with his mammy too and he loved them. Showers with mammy were a little different than with daddy though. There were certain things he loved and one thing he didn't particularly like. He never told me this, of course. He never wanted to hurt my feelings, God love him, and so just confided in his mammy instead. You see Barbara would always place Craig's jam-jams on the radiator before they got in the shower. When she was dressing him afterwards, Craig always appreciated how 'toasty' they were. He'd say, 'Oh Mammy, they're so warm,' and wriggle and giggle with satisfaction.

One day, after one such shower with Barbara, Craig asked her 'Why doesn't Daddy warm my jam-jams like you do?' Barbara laughed and told him that she'd say it to me—in a roundabout way of course. While he was on the topic he mentioned to his mammy that I never put his socks on right either and asked her to show me how. I apparently had a terrible habit of not pulling the socks up evenly on his ankles, so that the upper parts were scrunched up. Barbara reassured him that she'd make sure I did a better job in future.

However, there was one thing that Craig didn't like about having showers with his mammy. As Barbara recalls, Craig's reason for this was a great one: He told her he was afraid of touching off her 'hairy thing!' It seems that the presence of this was not to his liking. He didn't mind seeing his mammy's boobies mind you, just not the midriff Mohawk!

———

Another fantastic shower story comes to mind now which is definitely worth a mention. One night, as normal, we were in the shower when Craig began to cry uncontrollably. 'What's wrong?' I said. 'What happened?' I got the shock of my life hearing him crying like that. I didn't know what had happened, whether he'd hurt himself or not.

'I'm sorry, Daddy,' he cried. 'I was only trying to fart . . . I didn't mean to do it.'

I looked down and could see a small turd floating near his ankles and I started to laugh hysterically.

'Oh Jesus let me out, LET ME OUT!' Craig cried frantically as he danced his little hooves away from the approaching unit of menace below him and fast towards the shower door. He was petrified of *it* touching him. He pulled over the door and jumped outside.

'You're all right, Craig,' I said, trying desperately not to laugh so much at his plight. 'Don't worry about it. It's only pooh. Look, I'll get rid of it!' I reached down and scooped it up in my hand and walked out past Craig to the loo and dropped it in.

'I'm sorry,' Craig said again, 'it was just an accident.' He looked up at me and then we both got back into the shower. Inside, we started to laugh at how funny it was. After a while Craig said, 'I can't believe you picked up my pooh!'

Among the many things that I loved about Craig was his mischief and his cheeky devilment. Even shower time could not escape his impish ways. For instance, I can never forget the time Craig trapped me in the shower and froze me with the cold water. We were in the shower together and I was rinsing the shampoo out of my hair. Just as I finished this I opened my eyes and could see that Craig had moved away from his normal corner and to the corner beside the shower door handle. 'What are you doing?' I asked, innocently.

'Nothing,' was Craig's reply as he just stood stock still and began to smirk.

I knew at once there was something afoot. I knew that look too well. Then it hit me. I turned around rapidly and looked at the power switch on the shower. *It was off!* I nearly died. You see the thing about our shower back then was that it was slightly faulty. Whenever the power switch was turned off, it always took a further few minutes for the water to actually stop running. But well before the water would stop running, it would lose its heat. In fact, about ten to fifteen seconds after the shower being turned off the water would become icy cold. As soon I witnessed the *Off* position the daggers came. The icy water began to pour over me. I lost my breath as I moved to get out of the shower but Craig stood there blocking me. He laughed hysterically, but stood firmly, as I shouted at him to move out of the way. I was completely trapped. I reached around frantically to grab the nozzle from its placement and take the pain away. I looked at Craig then and pressed my hand against the shower door. 'Now you're trapped, Craig!' I said. But he just looked at me.

'Go on so,' he said. 'I don't care!'

And he didn't. I knew the cold water didn't bother him. After all the other previous showers we'd had together Craig would always stay behind and wait for the water to turn cold. He'd dare himself to do it and would stay there under the icy water until it stopped. When he'd get out, he'd have a big red face and an even bigger smile. 'You're a mad man, Craig,' is what I'd always say to him before drying him off.

So Craig knew my weakness and he got me. Another time he got me was almost worse than the cold shower. We had just finished our shower and were drying ourselves outside. We always had our shower in the en suite of the main bedroom and it was the tiniest en suite in the world. There was just room for the shower, a sink, and the toilet. Nothing more. So there we stood cramped up together trying to get dry as quickly as we could. I would always dry Craig first and then myself and this time was no different. I was standing at full height after drying Craig and was facing the door as I vigorously began drying my head and upper body. Then, out of nowhere, an icy knife ran across my lower back. The cold of it was incredible. It stole my breath, forcing my shoulders to hunch up, my neck to shorten, and my calves to tighten and leave me in a tippy toed stance as I fought to turn around. There stood Craig. He had his right hand cupped under the sink's cold tap, and it filled with more cruel water. Before I got to say anything he threw it on me. It took my breath again and I was so unbelievably shocked that Craig successfully got a third attack in too. I just about managed to grab his wrist in time and prevent the fourth from leaving his hand. But the laughter that exploded from Craig's face was simply marvellous. He thought it was the funniest thing he'd ever seen in his life and just couldn't stop himself. I remember that laugh so well.

This went on to become a recurring threat between us as the years went by: a kind of post-shower warfare. Neither of us would dare leave the other out of our sight when it came to drying. Invariably though at times we'd forget. Usually it would be me who'd be lost in my own world of thoughts, causing Craig to pounce on the opportunity and get me good. Other times it would be Craig who'd forget. I remember one such time cupping both my hands together and filling them to the top before emptying the whole lot over his head. He was so angry with me it was hilarious.

A new aspect that developed later on and became incorporated briefly into our evening shower routine was exercise. I'd decided that I was going to do a five-minute workout each evening just before I'd get into the shower. I started this first by heading upstairs a couple of minutes before Craig, getting in the nip and doing some floor exercises out in the landing. I wanted to do some press-ups, sit-ups and some other bits and pieces. When I'd finish I'd shout downstairs to Craig to come up and have his shower.

One evening though, only a few days after I'd started this routine, I was in the middle of my exercise when Craig's face appeared looking over the top of the stairs. 'What are ye doing?' he asked, a strange look on his face as he took in the naked monstrosity before him. I told him about my new exercise routine and in an instant he was in the nip too and lying down beside me mimicking my every action. From that moment, my exercise routine became *our* exercise routine. Craig wanted big muscles. It was as simple as that. It was funny actually. After every 'session' Craig would flex his biceps and get me to feel them to verify they were getting bigger and stronger—which I of course assured him were. I can still see Craig now as we both lay on our backs in the landing doing bicycle kicks, and how he said, after I'd stopped kicking through exhaustion, 'I don't need to stop, Daddy. I'm so strong I could go on forever,' whilst kicking even more furiously to make his point.

So this floor workout became an everyday routine for us, followed by the rewarding shower afterwards. Craig was really into it. He loved the idea of being a strong rugby player and even mentioned a desire to be a Chippendale no less. So he really took his exercises seriously. One night, however, we were late coming home and after racing to strip, Craig jumped straight into the shower. I had turned it on and we'd both clearly forgotten about the exercises. I ran out to the hotpress to grab some towels and it was only then that it hit me. In a flash I dropped to the floor and started to do some of the routines as fast as I could. As I lay there on my back, in the middle of some bicycle kicks, I got a strange feeling. Then I got the shock of my life. 'I knew it!! . . . I knew you were out here without me!!' Craig was standing over me, soaking wet and dripping water all over my startled head. I was taken aback. I moved to get up and fumbled my words like some guilty wrongdoer caught out doing a mischievous deed. 'Craig I . . . I forgot too . . . I just . . . I was getting the towels and . . .'

'No!' Craig interrupted, as he turned and stormed his way to the shower. 'It's not fair. I wanted to do my exercises too and you did them without me.'

He was so annoyed with me. I followed him into the shower and told him I was sorry and then promised him that we'd have a longer bedtime story to make amends. This did the trick, thankfully, and he was happy again. As I showered I reflected on how he must have so quietly, and with great stealth, climbed out of the shower to catch me. He must have been in the shower and then remembered the exercises. Immediately he must have wondered whether my absence meant I was out there—sin of all sins—doing the workout *without him*. But that image of Craig standing over me, so wronged, so righteous, is burned eternally into my mind now.

These are all such wonderful, treasured memories to have and all from something as commonplace and routine as having a shower. It really is the little things that mean so much in the end.

Craig loved adventure. He had a wonderful sense of excitement about doing something new and different. He embraced the unknown with enthusiasm and optimism. Like the time we were in Dunnes Stores and we happened upon a cheap and cheerful little two-man tent . . .

Camping in the Garden

The tent was assembled in the store and Craig rushed over and ran inside. He smiled and laughed as he poked his head back out and said, 'I wish I had one of these.' The subtle ways of children, eh!

So with that I got on my knees and joined him inside for a look and feel of how good it was. It was one of those easily assembled tents (which I very much liked) and was quite spacious inside. I checked the price and at €20 it was a bargain. *I'm going to buy this*, I thought. I told Craig and he was over the moon.

'Are you really?' he asked with a grin alive on his face. 'Ohhhh yesssss! . . . I can't believe it. Are we going to go camping then?'

'First things first, Craig. Let me buy it,' I answered.

I bought the tent and later that evening, as it was a fine summer's day, I told Craig that we were going to be camping in the back garden that night.

'ARE WE?' he shouted.

'Yep. Now c'mon and help me put it up.' Craig had no difficulty helping me and between me, him and his mammy we got the tent up in a matter of minutes. Craig jumped inside and thought it was so cool that we'd be sleeping outside. His excitement was infectious and I found myself really looking forward to the night's adventure ahead.

Later that evening Barbara got us some duvets and pillows and we fetched our sleeping beds to make up our camp for the night. We waited until bedtime, which was late for Craig in this instance, before heading out. We watched some stuff on the TV and ate junk food as part of our 'pre-camping' celebrations and all evening I fought off questions from Craig of 'When are we going out?' When it actually began to get dark enough we made our way outside and climbed inside to the relative safety the tent provided. I brought a torch with me too and this proved very useful later for setting the mood.

It was a cool evening outside so it felt wonderfully cosy to get all snuggled up into our sleeping bags. Just as we lay there in our sleeping bags I said to Craig, 'Let's tell some ghost stories,' to which he responded by sitting upright and saying 'Yeeeeaaaaah.' But just as I looked at Craig, getting ready to start some beastly tale, his big wide eyes and beaming smile gave way to a long yelping noise as his excitement got the better of him. He followed this with the words 'I'm just so happy!' as he beamed those little white teeth of his right in my face. I had to laugh at the intensity of Craig's happiness: he was jittering with joy. It was as if the prospect of ghost stories had exploded his joy out of control. It was infectious, though. God, it was so wonderful for me to see Craig in that state of joy.

Just then I turned the torch on and began to speak of ghouls and monsters and *The People of the Hedge*. We actually had a hedge that ran just behind our garden wall and stretched all around the border of our estate. I figured that some terror lurking within it might prove more of a tangible threat than other unspeakable terrors lurking in some distant graveyard somewhere. Naturally I of course reminded Craig of that hedge nearby and so every bird or cat that moved spoke of the most horrendous impending doom. We had been taking turns telling ghost stories up to that point but after hearing *The People of the Hedge* Craig decided he didn't want any more. So that ended that. We'd been telling them for a long while anyway so it was time to roll over and get some sleep.

I of course couldn't resist the old 'What was that?' routine every now and again. It worked a treat as always but ultimately it backfired on me. Craig had become so anxious that I think if he were capable of climbing into my skin he would have done so. He buried himself in beside me as he tried to sleep and feel safe. But you see I'm one of those people who generally need space when they sleep and so the idea of someone being right under my chin wasn't exactly conducive to my getting any sleep. It wasn't that bad, though. It was a cold evening and the extra heat, for once, was tolerable . . . Our first night of camping together.

I remember well one early Saturday morning when Craig, who was about four at the time, made his usual trek to our bed. As was always the case he'd stand at my side of the bed and wait for me to pull down the duvet before climbing over and lying between me and his mammy. But what proceeded to happen next was my witnessing of Craig's first ever Freudian slip . . .

Super Duper Sumo

On this particular morning he sat up between us playing with some toy cars. I didn't mind in the slightest. I was lying on my side, facing away from him as he drove the cars up and down my shoulders and back—a perfectly relaxing morning massage that I always welcomed. As I lay there just about to drift into a coma, Craig ran one of the cars along the side of my belly. As I was sleeping almost naked I could feel every motion of the cars as they moved along my side. However, in this particular instance I was sucked out of my coma as I listened to the tune Craig was humming while he moved the cars across my gut. I recognised it . . . and I laughed. It was the theme music to a cartoon that Craig often watched—*Super Duper Sumo*. It hit me that Craig was looking at my naked stomach and subconsciously had associated it with a sumo. I turned and looked at him:

'Are you singing *Super Duper Sumo*?'

Craig looked puzzled and then said 'Yeah.'

'Ye little fecker ye . . . you think I'm a sumo . . .' I said, astonished but laughing.

Craig burst his sides giggling when he realised I was right. He was surprised himself. Barbara didn't recognise the tune, but when she heard our chat and Craig's laughing we all ended up in tears that morning. A small but important memory . . .

Craig's inquisitive mind was something that I was very much used to but occasionally it shocked even me. I remember one cold afternoon in particular when Craig and myself were in the sitting room. Craig was four at the time, not that you'd think it . . .

Daddy . . . Where Do People Come From?

Craig was sitting on the sofa playing with his Yu-gi-oh cards while I sat in the armchair opposite reading the newspaper. As I was reading I could still see Craig in my periphery, looking down at his cards and shuffling through them as he always did. This was very much the scene until at one point, as I turned the page, I chanced a glance over at him. He was no longer shuffling the cards; instead his gaze was fixed forward to the fire burning in the grate. I thought nothing of it and carried on reading as before. But then Craig spoke:

'Daddy . . . where do people come from?' he asked, as I peered to the left of my paper and right at him.

What a bloody good question! I thought to myself. I remember swallowing, bracing myself to give some credible answer, but then Craig elaborated.

'I mean, I know I came from mammy's belly . . . and that she came from her mammy's belly . . . but where did the first person come from?' he said, looking right at me. 'Did they just come up out of the ground or something?'

I looked at him, raised my eyebrows, and blew an *I'm stumped* out-breath as I pondered how I was possibly going to answer that one.

'D'ye know what, Craig?' I said, being as honest as I could. 'That's the biggest question in the world . . . and nobody really knows the true answer.'

With that Craig simply made a *hmmm* expression and then turned back to his cards. I remember looking at him and wondering how a four-year-old boy could possibly be thinking such deep thoughts. But then that was our Craig . . .

Craig could have an incredibly stubborn streak, there's no denying it. I believe it went hand in hand with that sense of justice of his—what was right and what was wrong. I can still see that wonderfully expressive face of his frowning in the belief he was being hard done by. His brow would furrow and the arms would fold—he was letting us know. But sometimes, just sometimes, Craig would get the last laugh . . .

He Who Laughs Last . . .

There were countless times when Barbara and I would find ourselves in some pottery or craft shop telling Craig to 'Look, don't touch!' or 'Hands in the pockets, Craig!' only to catch him touching everything we'd just touched. He'd follow us around the shop and watch us picking up various pieces of interest and then place them back. That's when he'd strike. As soon as we'd turn he'd reach out and touch it. Furthermore he'd keep doing it until he was brave enough to do it in full view. 'Craig! . . . Don't touch that!' we'd say, terrified that he'd drop it.

'But you touched it!' he'd say, fully expecting the scorn and now ready for battle. 'It's not fair! Why is it always just me?' He'd be so angry, so righteous.

We'd get locked into a battle of words until finally we'd be forced to pull rank. All his sturdy arguments of 'But you could drop it too!'

and 'I am just as careful as you!' would be rebutted with our final, ruthless retort of 'Do as you're told!' Craig hated that. The eyebrows would pull in, the lips would purse and with nostrils flared he'd move away in disgust muttering 'It's not bloody fair!' He'd disappear to another side of the shop—as far away from us as he could—and loiter there until we had to go. We'd leave him to it too. No doubt he was touching things with gusto while out of sight but we'd let him off to cool down. Occasionally I or Barbara would turn around to see where he was, only to see half of his face emerging from behind a corner, the mother of all skulks beaming back at us.

On one occasion he did just this and so I stuck my tongue out at him—to lighten the mood. I remember seeing the chink in his armour as a grin appeared—reluctantly—in response. The head swiftly disappeared behind the corner in furious retreat at that point. I knew he was annoyed at letting his guard down so I just kept browsing with Barbara in the shop. A minute or so later I turned to see him standing in the spot again, his head now more in view than before. He was grinning, but this time he was the instigator of it. I smiled at him, knowing that the air had been cleared. But I also remember how the smile on my face vanished in an instant as the delayed reaction of my brain finally took in the ornament that he was holding against his belly. *The cheek of him*; 'Crraaaiiiig! . . .'

Yep, he certainly did have a bit of a stubborn streak, that's for sure. On another occasion, the details of which escape me now, we sent Craig to his room for being bold. It wasn't something we were used to doing with Craig, so whatever the reason, it must have been significant. Anyway, he marched up to his room and stayed there. I'm not sure how long we left him up there, but it was long enough as far as we were concerned. Barbara had made some dinner so I walked out to the hall, looked up towards the landing and called up, 'Craig . . . you can come down now.'

Silence.

'Craig, come down . . . your dinner's ready!' I repeated, my voice more intense this time.

'Nnnooooo! . . . I'm not wanted down there . . .' he finally shouted, obviously recoiling from the patronising nature of how he was being handled.

When I heard this I grinned to myself. His sense of being wronged was so intense and his stubbornness so strong. 'It's up to you; your dinner's only going to get cold,' I said as I walked back into the kitchen. Barbara was smiling at how strong-willed he was.

'You'd think we were the ones who had been bold,' Barbara said as she began getting ready to dish up.

A minute or so later I heard the call. 'Daadddy!' Craig shouted down, his voice softer now, calmer.

'Yeahh?' I called back up, sensing his surrender.

'A bird is after flying into my window,' he said.

I couldn't quite believe what I was hearing, and ran up the stairs to his room. Craig was standing at the window looking out to the estate. 'What did you say?' I asked.

He kept staring out as he repeated the same curious message—'A bird just flew towards me and hit the window . . . I think he's dead.'

This was a most unexpected conversation and so I raced back downstairs to check outside the front door. I half believed he was winding me up. But sure enough, there in front of the door step, a dead starling lay on the ground—blood coming out of his beak and his tongue hanging to one side. I remember shaking my head with complete disbelief. I felt sorry for the little bird and removed it from the step. When I was finished I laughingly imagined Craig as some Omen child commanding the hapless starling to a Kamikaze end and therein purging himself of the frustration he was feeling. Ah yes it made me laugh. I went back up to Craig, who was still in his room, and he was smiling now as he explained how he'd gotten such a fright as the bird kept coming towards the window and then finally crashed into it. We laughed together and then Craig finally came down for his dinner . . . at last!

Like most parents, I'm sure, Barbara and I when going to bed each night would ritually check on Craig in his room. It's just something you do. Anyway there are two particular occasions that come to mind immediately when I think of this little practice. They stand out because they didn't follow the normal routine of this usually predictable night time observance . . .

Who Goes There?

On the first occasion, I found myself creeping upstairs at about 10.30 p.m. to get something. I wasn't going to bed, just fetching something or other. Craig had been in bed well over two hours at this stage and I knew he was asleep. After I got what I was looking for I passed his room on my way to the stairs. As always the door was wide open to allow the light from the hall to shine into the darkness. Just as I was about go past the room I decided I'd have a quick check on him, but instead of going in I thought I'd just look through the gap between the door and the frame. Craig's bed was right behind the door with his head nearest the door frame end. The room inside was too dark, and the light behind me made it difficult to focus as I peeked through. The part of the room where Craig was sleeping was the darkest because it was within the shadow of the door. So there I stood, looking through the thin gap to the spot where I knew Craig's head should be. My eyes shifted and wandered slightly, and I had to frame my gaze with both hands to eliminate stray light coming into my periphery. It took longer than expected for my eyes to adapt to the darkness within but then I got a shock. As I finally made out the covers and pillow, I moved my gaze to where Craig's head was. Two blue eyes were staring right back at me from the darkness.

Just at that moment, the two eyes spoke, simply asking 'What?'— no doubt wondering what the hell I was up to. I laughed, wondering how long he'd been watching me, waiting for our eyes to meet. It was a peculiar, funny moment that has stuck with me.

The next occasion was something similar but this time I was actually going to bed. It was about 11.30 p.m. I walked into Craig's room and stood at the handle of his door looking down on him as he slept. I stood there for a while, just watching him, trying to hear him breathe or see his chest rise and fall. I couldn't leave until I was sure he was alive—a typical parental attitude no doubt. Anyway I don't know how long I was standing there, maybe ten seconds, but as I looked at him Craig just flashed his eyes open and looked back. He screamed with the fright of seeing me, which caused me to scream right back in return. It was a double shock and Craig wasn't happy.

'What are you doing standing there?' he quizzed, and rightly too.

'I thought you were asleep!'

'I was . . . What are you doing?' I hadn't answered his question.

I told him that mammy and I checked on him every night like that, but usually he was fast asleep.

'Yeah, well, you're after scaring me now,' he scowled, followed immediately by 'You may get in beside me for a few minutes now—until I go back to sleep.'

Craig always knew how to turn a situation around . . . to suit *him*.

Barbara told me—only recently in fact—about a little secret she and Craig shared. It happened a few years back and I knew nothing about it.

The Secret Loan

It was a Friday and as normal Barbara was off that day. Ordinarily Fridays were for housework but on this particular Friday Barbara found herself not quite in the mood. I was at work as usual but I wouldn't be coming back that night. I was heading to a workmate's stag party in Kilkenny; a rare night out for me and I was looking forward to it.

Back at home Barbara realised she was skint, but really wanted to do something different with the day. The thoughts of housework just sickened her and Craig too was looking to go somewhere and get out of the house.

'But I've no money, darling,' Barbara said to Craig after he asked to go out.

'You could get a loan in the Credit Union,' Craig offered out of nowhere.

Barbara looked at him with a mixture of astonishment and some consideration for his idea. Craig knew we'd been to the Credit Union before to get loans at Christmas so, in his eyes, *no money* was simply solved by a visit to the magical place called the Credit Union. *Hey Presto, problem solved.*

Barbara's first thought was *No*. She couldn't justify a loan on a whim. She looked at Craig and he stared back up.

'I can't do that, darling,' she said, unconvinced.

'C'mon . . . we can go to Wexford!' he continued.

'No, I can't!'

'You can buy a top!' Craig was pushing the right buttons now.

Barbara thought about it—not for long, mind you—and then said *Well, why not!* She and Craig marched up to the Credit Union and up the stairs to see about the loan. They met with a lady and sat across from her. Before anything else got underway Craig just blurted out 'Will you give my mammy money?' The lady just laughed as Craig flashed his adorable little dimples at her. It worked though. They got a loan for €150—just for the day. But there was a caveat: *We can't tell Daddy.* This was paramount and Craig understood completely. It was their little secret.

So, €150 the richer, their first port of call that day was to go and get a pizza in the restaurant in Gorey. Craig proceeded to order a huge Margheritta pizza and then only eat two slices: sheer extravagance. Barbara had something nice herself and when all was finished they drove down to Wexford. As per Craig's suggestion Barbara bought herself that nice top, with Craig of course getting a toy into the bargain. They spent a lovely time together and before they eventually left they even stopped in for a cup of tea and some cake. It had been a very successful, treasured day indeed . . . and I never ever found out about that loan until it came to writing this book.

Getting to meet President McAleese in Áras an Uachtaráin certainly stands out as a very special day in our lives and especially Craig's. Thanks to my sister Melanie, who works in Áras an Uachtaráin, we got this once-in-a-lifetime opportunity to meet and stand for a photograph with the President and her husband, Dr Martin McAleese, during Christmas 2005 . . .

Meeting the President

Officially it was 'The Christmas Tree lighting ceremony' with any number of guests traditionally invited to this annual event. This year, thanks to Mel, we were on the guest list and boy, were we looking forward to it. It was such an honour to be in attendance in this historic place and in the presence of the President. We were particularly delighted for Craig, who, although completely unfazed by the significance of the event, was very excited about 'going to the president's house'. He had already told people in his class and was feeling very special indeed.

On the day itself we drove up to Áras an Uachtaráin and met up with Mel who greeted us outside. Along with Craig, Barbara and myself, Mel had invited my parents and Uncle Mike and Aunt Marie. We all followed Mel's lead and entered the prestigious building in tow. It was a wonderful feeling as we walked through those doors and into a place that very few people get to see. We all felt overwhelmingly grateful to Mel for giving us this rare opportunity, knowing as we did that not one of us would be there were it not for her.

The sense of history as we walked down the corridors and into different rooms was incredible. It oozed from every wall and archway and with every passing second I felt more and more honoured to be there. Barbara and I looked at each other and then down at Craig and were so chuffed for him—so young and to be meeting the President. Because of the day that was in it, Santa was present too and Craig didn't hesitate in taking his turn in meeting him. He received a small gift and told Santa what he wanted for Christmas before making his way back to us. He was delighted.

Eventually the time came to meet the President and so we made our way to the designated area. Before long we were in the surreal position of standing with President McAleese and Dr McAleese, shaking hands and posing for photographs. It was fantastic. The President said a few words to Craig, who cheekily smiled up at her and spoke back, and after all the photos were taken we quietly moved out to the main reception area. It was only when we left the President that we realised Craig had been holding a balloon sword in his hand, now immortalised in every presidential photo we were in.

In the main reception area people were gathering and nibbling on food. Just then Ryan Tubridy walked into the room and, although we tried not to, we found ourselves eyeballing him as different people came up and spoke with him and stood for pictures. As far as I can recall my father nabbed him too and both he and my mother got in a picture with him. It was a strange moment within a very unusual day.

Before long President McAleese came out and addressed the room of assembled guests. A wonderful, eloquent speaker as always, she thanked everyone for coming and then officially marked the lighting of the huge Christmas tree which was actually outside on the grounds of Áras an Uachtaráin—ordinarily the ceremony was conducted outside but with such bad weather that couldn't happen.

All in all we spent a couple of hours there, with Mel even giving us a guided tour of the office area. We actually got to meet a colleague of Mel's—the speechwriter, I believe—who was very welcoming and kind to us. He was particularly nice to Craig and even tried to show him how to use a kind of boomerang toy, which didn't work. Craig gave it a lash all right but as soon as it didn't return he was done with it.

A few weeks after this special meeting we received copies of the photos taken, all signed, 'Best Wishes, President McAleese.' They were beautiful and treasured, but there—like a sore thumb—was that balloon sword. We laughed and thought no more of it. It didn't matter.

However, just as I was sitting to write this particular account for the book I looked up at the picture in question which happened to be hanging on the wall in front of my desk. I stared at it for ages—the mischievous smile on Craig's face and the balloon in hand—and I grinned. The balloon, as luck would have it, was exactly the same shade of pinky-purple as Mary's matching lipstick, suit and shoes. How fortuitous indeed. . . . Trust the little scamp to accessorise with such fashion consciousness.

Most people who knew Craig would agree that he was not your average youngster. There was something of the 'little man' about him. Talking with Craig it was easy to forget sometimes just how young he was . . .

Our Little Man

My father can certainly attest to Craig's maturity: the many drives they shared together were always accompanied by fascinating, quality banter. He always remarked on how good Craig's company really was; admitting that when he spoke to Craig it was the very same as if he were with an adult.

And my mother was the same. She was always struck by Craig's honesty, thoughtfulness and understanding, the level of which belied his young years. But she always remembers so fondly the very first moment that Craig came to see her cottage. Craig had walked around it, taking it all in and getting a feel for it before simply turning and saying 'This is a grand little cottage you have here, Nana!'—a right little man altogether. Although just to show he was still very much the little boy he then proceeded to play a prank on her. Herself and Craig were over near her garage, with my mother about to water the plants. It was a beautiful hot summer's day and my mother asked Craig to turn the tap on and hand her the hose. All of a sudden there were screams. Craig had done exactly what she asked, but then decided to water his Nana—and not the flowers.

Even in school the teacher's assistant, Adrienne, who sat beside him, would find herself frequently opening up to Craig about things in her life that she normally wouldn't talk about to any other child (or adult for that matter). Craig had that way about him. He was a great listener: he did actually listen to what you were saying and I suppose that in itself is a rarity for most of us.

Craig was considerate of others' feelings too. Barbara's mother remembers fondly the night she looked after him while we all attended his benefit night in Enniscorthy. This had been organised for Craig by Barbara's brother Shane and his wife Tracey. That night they had such fun together, messing and chatting away and with Craig eating everything around him. Eventually though, towards the end of the night she and Craig moved and sat together on the couch. Craig was feeling sleepy. He was on heavy medication at the time and that, coupled with the feast he'd gorged on, had left him feeling completely drained by the end of the night. While sitting there on the couch, with his Nana beside him, he looked up at her and spoke. 'Nana, will you be ok on your own if I fall asleep?' . . . even then he was thinking of another and not himself.

We have lovely video footage, which I've watched a few times since Craig passed, of a Nativity play he was part of when he was at Higgy's House Montessori. I remember at the time how wonderful it was to watch Craig being 'The Narrator' as all the other children played their little parts. We had practised his lines every night at bedtime for about two weeks before the big performance. But on the day Craig was a real trooper. He stood front and left of stage with his two hands behind his back and rocking back and forth from heel to toe. He'd remind you of an old man or 'Dinny' from Glenroe. While there was a frenzy of activity behind him, he'd occasionally look in and, pointing the way, instruct the other little actors on where they needed to be. He was the embodiment of calm, delivering his lines and then rocking on the spot. At one point during the performance he even looked right at my camera and, with a nod of the head, gave a confident wink. It was priceless. There wasn't a worry in his head. It was all under control. But he actually became too confident in the end. A hand—an adult hand, that is—appeared from behind 'the curtain' tapping him—prompting him—to say his line. He'd become so relaxed he'd forgotten about his participation in the play.

But for his young years—those very few years—he displayed a maturity of manner and mind which far exceeded them. He truly was our 'Little Man'.

Chapter 4

Better Times

2005 began with the constant threat of redundancy looming over my head. Craig was only four and a half. But *where* I worked, although ridiculously far away, fitted in delicately with how Barbara, Craig and myself commuted every morning. Over the years our daily commute was arranged like a well-oiled machine and so my moving to another company elsewhere in Dublin would mean a disastrous change to everything. It would mean upheaval for all of us and inevitably a worsening in our quality of life. It was this fact above all that niggled away at me as the year moved forward.

I never feared *not* getting another job, just *where* that job would be. In the five years living and commuting from Gorey there was no improvement whatsoever in the job scene in the Wexford/Wicklow area for someone in my position. It was a bleak truth to face— knowing that my advancing career and all the experience, training and qualifications garnered served only to further cement my dependence on working in the Dublin area and a life of impossible commutes: a life of diminished family time and foreseen regret. And there certainly was no way we were ever going to be in a position to afford moving closer to Dublin. It simply wasn't an option. But even more important than that was how much we, as a family, enjoyed living in Gorey. We had made it our home in those years and we were lining Craig up to begin his schooling down there that year. I always held the belief that people should change their job to suit their life, not change their life to suit their job.

But the dark cloud of redundancy, for all the turmoil it promised, was also a double-edged sword. I can honestly admit that I was far from being entirely displeased by the notion of losing that job. In a weird and wonderful way it offered hope of change. Our family life had suffered for years at the hand of—and I have to be honest—my job. I had tried so often over the preceding years to find work closer to home but always failed. We were trapped by the road I had taken. So the potential for redundancy simultaneously scared and elevated me. I revelled in the latent opportunity that had walked into my life. A redundancy would force my hand and perhaps unearth some sequence of events which could possibly lead (oh joy of joys!) to my finding a completely different job and a career closer to home. This charged one half of my mind with a zeal that only the unknown can offer. In many ways I have always been an optimist in life and so the excitement I felt at possible changes to the status quo often outweighed the inherent fears I harboured. Barbara was more of a pessimist—although she would say a realist—and so she wore the garment of fear and worry for both of us.

Amongst the tumult of that opening year was the preparation for Craig's transition from a life in Bray, to a life in Gorey. He would be starting school that year and so no more would he be joining us on our treks. But first we had to register Craig in a school. In fact the day I brought Craig in for registration was very memorable indeed.

God he was as cool as a cucumber as he sat down in that office across from the teacher. The whole setup had the feeling of an interview, with the teacher on one side of the desk and Craig on the other. I was almost like a bystander as she proceeded to chat away with Craig. I smiled all the way through it too. I was just so proud of how he handled himself. He was so calm and confident, totally unfazed by speaking with this adult and authority figure. He sat upright on a large green padded chair and presented himself with such honesty and beautiful charisma. I'm not sure what the other children's backgrounds were—whether they'd been in crèches/Montessoris or not—but Craig was so easy with himself in that situation.

Actually, before we ever went into the office I remember the chaos and noise outside in the corridor. Boisterous and excited kiddies filled the corridor, while sulkers and screamers filled the air. In among it all sat Craig. He was so eager yet so relaxed. One boy walked up to him and after saying 'Hello' just turned around and walked off. I can still see Craig's face now as he looked up at me with a smile and a delighted 'What was that about?' expression on his face. But it was just his composure that I was so impressed with. It was like the corridor was filled with wild animals while Craig was domesticated. I was worried he was nervous, but then, out of the blue, he just got up. He coolly walked over to two boys and they talked. Craig was a big chap, so he towered over the other two but they all seemed to mingle quite well. It was great to see. It brought some relief, I can tell you. I knew then that Craig was going to be ok.

But in the office Craig really shone. He answered all the questions politely and spoke with a freedom from anxiety that most of the rest of us will never have in our lives. He even asked the teacher a question of his own. I cannot remember what it was, but it certainly did please her. She smiled and looked at me with raised eyebrows saying 'He's a great fella, isn't he. Not a bother on him at all.' Craig loved that. He looked right over at me then and flashed his little dimples. And I was proud. I was exceptionally proud, I can tell you. When we were finished and we made our way to the door, the teacher just turned and said it again to me—'He's a great chap, isn't he? I just can't get over how mature he is. You wouldn't think he was that age at all.' It was lovely to hear and to know Craig had made such an impression.

———

On 11 September 2005, Barbara received a call that absolutely devastated her. We were at home in Gorey at the time and Barbara was in the kitchen. On the other end, her brother Shane delivered the unthinkable news that her father had died. I can still see Barbara collapsing to the floor as those catastrophic words pulled the legs from under her. She let out a heart-rending cry as she fell to the floor. Watching, I knew. Craig was beside me and he was scared by what was happening. He didn't know why his mammy was so upset and kept pleading, 'Mammy, what's wrong, what's wrong?' but Barbara simply couldn't speak. I took Craig by my side and picked up the phone to speak with Shane. He confirmed to me what I already knew and after passing on my sympathies I turned to Craig.

'Your mammy's very upset because she was just told that her daddy—your granddad—has gone to heaven.' I knew I had to explain this to Craig.

'Nooooo!' Craig began to cry as the news overwhelmed him. 'Noooo . . . my granddad . . . Noooo!'

I hugged Craig and told him that his granddad was in a better place and that he was no longer in any pain. But Craig was so upset. He was also confused why his mammy wouldn't speak to him and kept asking me why she was mad at him. I reassured Craig that she wasn't angry with him and did my best to explain what she was going through, trying to minimise his pain and uncertainty in this most poignant and dreadful moment. I knew that his granddad dying was something we would need to discuss and help him deal with but I also needed to be there for Barbara.

The house, in the turn of a moment, was utter chaos. Emotions and tears filled our home and all sense of coherence and normality had gone. I tried to comfort Barbara but she was in deepest despair, unwilling to listen to anything outside the darker thoughts that now settled on her mind.

After a while Barbara received another call, from her mother, Breda, still in the hospital. She wanted Barbara to call down to the family home to sit with her brother Patrick. She didn't know how long she'd be and didn't want Patrick by himself in the house. So we agreed to go down but weren't looking forward to it. You see Patrick didn't know yet. Breda thought it best that we say nothing until she got home. She was afraid of how he would react and wanted to tell him herself. She wanted to be there for him.

We were incredibly anxious as we later arrived at the house, knowing that we'd have to keep the truth from Patrick. We hated being in that situation, and thought it so wrong to sit there chatting away as if everything was fine and normal. An hour or two passed before Breda and the rest of the family finally arrived home. As they came in through the back door, it was the sound of wailing that hit first. Sisters Sandra, Shirley and Tina, along with Breda had tears running down their faces. I had a sickening knot in my stomach as I watched Patrick look up from his seat to his mother who was crying and walking towards him. 'What is it, Mammy? What's wrong? How's Daddy?' he called out, knowing in his heart what his mother's tears implied. She told him. With that there was another outcry of emotion as Patrick was overpowered by this horrifying reality.

'Not Daddy,' he cried, 'Not Daddy . . . No!' It had hit him hard. Breda hugged into him, but he wriggled and swayed with the pain. He shook his head, fighting the reality that poured into his every sense, but which would not be ignored. It was then that Patrick realised that we had known the truth and hadn't told him.

'But Barbara didn't say anything,' he yelped, looking at his mother and feeling betrayed and confused. 'She knew and she said nothing!' he cried.

'I'm so sorry, Patrick,' Barbara cried in response. 'I was told not to say anything. I wanted to tell you but I couldn't.' Barbara was devastated seeing and hearing Patrick in such a state and feeling so guilty for having said nothing.

'Don't be angry at Barbara,' Breda said, looking at Patrick. 'It's not her fault. I told her to say nothing until I got back.'

The scene was horrific and one I can never forget. I sat there among a family destroyed. Tears, cries, sobs upon faces that told of unspeakable pain. I'd never known tragedy in my life; I had been spared it. But for this family, who sat crippled before me, tragedy was something that had called time and again. I thought how unfair it was that these people were being subjected to so much. *How much more could they take?*

After the tears came the many silences . . . and it was unbearable. We sat in the front room all hunched together and yet silence pervaded through the increasingly broken talk. Everyone was present and accounted for—in body that is. Minds, however, were adrift on seas of pain and memory. I watched as eyes gazed out, fixed upon nothing, scrutinising not a thing. They were the stares of the bewildered; words seemed redundant now. I could feel the heaviness in the air and yet it rested not on my shoulders but on those around me whose lives had been eternally altered and diminished. The husband, the father, the patriarch of this family was dead.

I mourned Paddy's passing and felt his loss too. He was a good man; a man whom I respected and admired greatly and who had always made me feel welcome. But what I felt was only a millionth of the monumental loss that this family had just suffered. I had known Paddy only briefly and yet his character was such that I always knew I was in the company of a good man. He had impressed upon me certain values that I now hold dear: his calmness; his *c'est la vie* attitude to those things that others would make monsters of. There was a burning intelligence and a quiet dignity there. He was a man who just got on with things and who left the drama and nonsense to the rest. He had no time for it. His was a clearer view, a higher perspective. He'd sit quietly on the bank while the rest flailed and floundered.

But some months after Paddy's death a strange thing happened. My father was driving along the N11 with Craig when without any warning Craig began to cry hysterically. 'I miss my granddad!' he wept, putting his hands over his face to hide the tears.

My father was shocked and quickly looked at him.

'I wish I was dead too so I can be with him,' he continued to cry.

'Ah Craig,' my father said, 'don't say that. We don't want you to die. We want you here, with us. Your granddad wouldn't want that either.' He tried his best to calm him. 'Your mammy and daddy, and all of us, would be so sad if you went away.'

'I just miss him so much,' Craig said, as he settled again and composed himself.

This little outbreak was so out of character for Craig and came completely out of nowhere. On reflection, and considering what was to come, that moment is all the more poignant now.

———

I remember well how, as the late spring, early summer months of 2006 rolled in, bringing with them some measure of fine weather, I was fortunate enough to spend much more quality outdoor time with Craig. Our lives up until that point had been so extraordinarily lacking in quality time that having it at all was a real novelty. I loved it. I'd leave work at 3 p.m. and sing all the way home to Gorey. That may sound like an exaggeration but I swear it's not. I'd listen to the radio while belting out a few numbers as I motored along. Nobody, except Barbara, could understand the complete joy I felt at being able to come home and spend that time with Craig. There was no price I could put on it.

During my time as a contractor to BT I felt like the luckiest man in the world. Myself and Jackie, a colleague and friend of mine from my Galileo days, had felt so exceptionally fortunate to have been scooped up by BT when leaving Galileo. It was such a perfect move for both of us, financially and time-wise. On top of that we couldn't have asked for a nicer bunch of people to work with. There was a great atmosphere among us all and the banter was top notch.

For me though working in BT represented much more than all that. As I'd drive home in the mid-afternoon each day I would thank the heavens for this period in my life. The lifestyle, the family time it afforded me was out of this world. I could never have hoped to find such an opportunity, yet there I'd be—arriving at my door at 4 p.m. after a full day's work. I would drive up through the estate and frequently see Craig with his friends, standing and chatting. He'd look around and see me and then immediately come running after the car. I can still see the image of him chasing full throttle in my rear-view mirror.

I'd pull into the driveway and climb out of the car just in time to brace myself as Craig hurtled towards me shouting 'Daaddddyyy' and then leaped into my arms. I loved it . . . and I never once took that for granted. To have someone love you that much and to be so happy to see you every day was so humbling. Every time he'd do it he'd make me feel so special and good about myself. I'd hug him strongly in return, holding him up in my arms and squeezing the life out of him. He'd give me that extraordinary welcome and then, quick as he came, was off to his mates again . . . simple as that, eh.

On one of those days just as I'd come in from work Craig came in with his football and asked me to come out and play with him. It was a particularly sunny day too so I grabbed my runners and shorts and headed out with him for a kick around . . .

Me & Craig v The Rest of the World (aka 'The Estate Kids')

It started off as normal, with just myself and Craig kicking the ball backwards and forwards and yappin' away about school and various wonderful nonsense. Then I made some small goals—only about a metre wide—so that we could play 'funny football'. This was a game that my brother Darren and I used to play when we were young. We'd set the goal size to be small and then we'd play one on one against each other. The small goal size prevented lazy long shots, and ensured plenty of tackling and skill. Invariably though this would reduce us to fits of giggles as all sorts of cheating and messing went on.

So Craig and I would play this very same game, laughing and giggling as I tormented him with occasional cheating. Sometimes I'd let Craig get past me and as I'd fall to the ground watch in hysterics as he ran with such intensity and focus and complete concentration, kicking the ball as he went until finally putting it through the two make-shift posts.

It makes me laugh now as I think of it. There was this one moment as we played where we were both a long way from the goals. We'd been chasing and falling over one another, just laughing with tired giddiness. But I remember, as we wrestled, how Craig had quickly broken away from me and made straight for the goals. He knew I'd given up and was not really pursuing him but still he went like a train, destined for glory. However, he hadn't counted on standing on the ball as he ran, which instantly threw him to the ground. I knew he was all right by the way he fell and more importantly by how quickly he got back up. As soon as he did I gave chase. I sprinted after him shouting loudly, and putting the fear of God in him. He was a good distance ahead of me but I knew I could catch him before he got to the goal. But man did he run. He ran like his life was at stake. I shouted louder and louder as I grew closer and I knew that Craig must have had shivers down his spine as he felt me getting closer. Just as I got right up to him, ready to lift him up off the ground, Craig toe-bogged the ball and we both watched as it sped forward in a straight line, going clear through the two posts. Well I'd never seen Craig so excited in his life. He leapt up and down on the spot with both arms raised high into the air. It was the sweetest victory. I don't think he believed he'd get it. I in the meantime had collapsed onto the ground after my Olympic sprint and laughed as I clapped my hands in approval.

'Well done . . . ye little fecker ye!' I said, through what little breath I had left. Then Craig who was still jumping for joy came running towards me and jumped into the air, landing perfectly on top of me and giggling into my face. The victory was his and he loved it.

Soon after this a couple of kids came along to join us. They suggested we make teams and that we play against each other. These boys were about ten or eleven, I'd say, and so we agreed that it would be them against Craig and me. We set up our goals and began playing. We both had 'free' goalies so as to get a better game out of it. Craig was our goalkeeper and he took the job seriously. He defended well and I was too strong for the two lads. We were hammering them. In retrospect maybe I should have taken it a little easier on them but this was football and I wanted to win. Plus every time I scored Craig would leap into the air and shout 'Nice one, Daddy!' I was a sucker for the praise, I guess.

But then something strange happened. Over an impossibly short period of time more and more children began to appear on the green looking to join in. It was like something from the *Children of the Corn* as these kids kept coming from nowhere. Each time they would join forces with our opponent team and soon it became a massive contest with just me and Craig against 'The Rest of the World'. It was by no means an extravaganza of football but boy did we play our hearts out. I actually nearly did play my heart out: at about 300 bpm it was under fierce strain, I can assure you. The dedication and effort I put in was extraordinary. Christ, it felt like I was playing for my country, the amount of sheer commitment I displayed. And yet I was hopelessly unfit. Craig did a sterling job in goals and in coming out to help me. He'd shout from behind and run into spaces, while always controlling his goal area. But alas we were being overpowered by sheer numbers (of kids? . . . I know). I was fit to collapse. At seventeen and a half stone I'm sure I actually put my life at risk. I was trying to look good in front of Craig but I'm fairly certain my bulging, scaldy red eyes peering out against the backdrop of my big sweaty purple head and blue lips were about as far from 'looking good' as can be imagined.

It was around this time that I began to use my advantage. At my size, what I lacked in fitness I more than made up for in power and momentum. I began walking towards their goal, just pushing these pesky kids out of my path. As I did, I could hear Craig shouting 'Go on Daddy! Go on!' I ground my way through the mob of kids and I'm sure from the passer-by viewpoint it looked more like a rugby scrum. I moved relentlessly, stoically goal-ward. Forcefully I made my gains before finally hoofing the ball through their two jumpers. From about four metres out there really probably was no need for the 100 kph belt I'd given it, sending it almost clean out of the estate, but one had to be sure. Plus, of course, it gave me a chance to suck oxygen in before we started again.

I did this over and over again until we were almost level. Craig was cute enough too. At one stage he moved forward, ahead of the mob surrounding me, and waving his hands let me know he was there. Like

Moses parting the Red Sea I recall how I reached forward and pulled the kids apart before knocking the ball up to Craig who duly scored a neat little goal. It was a cracker.

We seemed to be playing for hours. I think we probably did too. All I know is that at some point I hit 'the wall' and started to feel sleepy. I knew I'd overdone it. I hadn't done any bloody exercise in years and now I was running on empty. My body had been stripped of all its reserves. Every vitamin and mineral I'd ever taken had been ripped from my system. All sugar reserves depleted, I grew heavy (heavier) and tired. My eyes began to blink longer than normal and I began to breathe deeply. I wanted to lie down and just kip. I was completely spent. The timing was perfect though because just about then Barbara came out and called us home for dinner. I was so relieved. We'd worked hard to get to level pegging and I knew I had nothing left to give. This way we got to leave with our heads held high (metaphorically of course for me . . . my head was either down between my knees gasping for air like a landed fish or sucking the life out of a Bricanyl inhaler for my asthma!). Yes, relieved is the word.

After dinner and a shower I remember sitting on the couch feeling like an exhausted and heavy hippo. The inertia was incredible. I sat there staring at the TV with my mouth wide open, and with dribble running down my chin(s). I didn't even have the energy to do a swallow. I was wrecked. Actually when it came to putting Craig to bed and reading him a story I decided to climb in beside him. I told him a story from my cosy horizontal position and as far as I can remember I think it involved something about being lost out in a cold and windy night and then finding a small, snug little hollow to get out of the storm and just sleep. As I told this story I found my own eyes beginning to close. Craig fell asleep rather quickly and I decided to stay there with him. I fell asleep for a while myself in fact. I had to force myself to get up and go back downstairs. It was terrible. I think I had a few things to do first, but once they were done I had an early night.

The next morning every muscle in my body was sore. I felt like I'd been placed in a bag and trampled by livestock. Even my mouth was sore—obviously from the strain of hoovering down lung-fulls of air into my shocked body. It was 6 a.m. as I drove to work, all buckled and battered, and all I could think was how Craig had asked 'Can we do the same again tomorrow?'

Of the many qualities Barbara and I admired about our Craig, his resolve probably impressed us most. Time and time again we'd see how his dogged persistence paid off . . .

Never Give Up

Although we lived in Gorey, Craig's daily life was pretty much entirely based in Bray. Up until shortly after he turned five, Craig's days were 7.40 a.m. to 6 p.m., Monday to Friday in Bray. Because of this he never really got a proper chance to play with or befriend the other boys and girls on our estate in Gorey. It was difficult when they all knew each other and he was just some kid who was around every now and again. We used to feel so sorry for him, and guilty: this was all down to us after all, not him.

I suppose I didn't really want to admit it to myself, but I was concerned. I was scared that Craig would find it difficult to make friends down home and would feel alienated as a result.

When Craig reached that age where he wanted to get out of the house on his own, we left him to it. We were anxious but eager to see how he'd fare. We were blessed by the fact that Craig was always so keen to get out and mix with other children. We didn't have to push or encourage him to go—he just went out the door.

It was usually quite late in the evening (when we returned from work) when Craig got his chance to get out. In those early attempts Craig would often come back after only a short ramble looking defeated. 'There's nobody around,' he'd say, before playing with some toys near the window, looking out. Other times he'd go out only to come flying back through the door ten minutes later, bawling his eyes out telling us what some of the kids had said to him. And kids certainly can be mean. It was very hard for us to witness this. We knew the kids out on the estate were all close and that Craig was really just a stranger trying to fit in. I despaired each time this happened, not knowing what to do—how to make it all better for him. Yes, we were angry with the other kids, but then kids are kids. All it takes is one to be mean and the rest can easily follow suit. Craig just needed time. Craig didn't have the time though, we thought, knowing that he was home so late in the evenings. We felt terrible for making this so hard on him.

So, we being utterly useless as parents in this regard, it was down to Craig to resolve this problem himself. Like I said, when Craig would come in the door crying 'They told me to go away!' or 'They told me to stop following them, to leave them alone,' we'd feel so incredibly heartbroken and powerless to help him. I'd silently curse myself for doing a job that caused all this. I'd hate myself and panic, thinking how the hell I can change it all. But neither I nor Barbara wanted to force them to play with him: that would do more harm than good. We simply had to stay out of it and just hope that things would improve.

Craig would eventually stop sobbing and yet still Barbara and I would look at each other knowing that we had failed him. We knew he was such a people person and that he got on with everyone, but in this instance we had orchestrated an impossible situation for him and he was suffering the consequence.

We'd sit there with our heads down, sighing and worrying about how he was going to get through all this, only to hear the door bang. We'd look up at each other and then out the front window and see Craig standing on the path. Here we were worrying about his fragility and how we were ever going to persuade him to get out again and yet he'd simply dried his tears, got up and walked straight back out the door.

The first time Craig did that we were immensely proud. He had shown such character. I remember looking out the sitting room window and seeing him standing back out on the road. He was alone but he was not giving up. He stood there, looking up the road to where the others were gathered, and slowly he'd begin to saunter back up. I was incredibly inspired by his strength of will and his gut determination . . . and so relieved too. Yet again he had made our job as parents that much easier. He took away the burden of resolution from us and sorted it out himself. We were so lucky that Craig had that inner resolve, the self-confidence and inner belief to keep at it. We don't know what we would have done otherwise. Were he weaker, more timid or less determined we'd have had an almighty task on our hands.

Many times he was faced with such scathing attacks by the other children and still he'd persist in going back. It was because of the irregular nature of when he got to meet up with them that he had to suffer these backlashes. The times he got out to see them were very few. As a result they were in their own little clique, leaving Craig to battle his way in each time.

There were several occasions when Craig came running into the house saying that one of the boys had kicked or punched him. This was a disturbing development and one that had to be acted upon. Barbara confronted the child in question and gave him a good telling off, but was surprised at his size. Craig was a big chap and this little fella was no match for him. Craig was a big softy really. He was never one for fighting and certainly wasn't violent. But after this happened a few times, with Craig coming in the door crying, yet again because of the same fella hitting him, we had to change our tack. There was no sense in us constantly fighting Craig's battles for him and nor would that benefit him in the long run. So, we told Craig that he was going to have to stand up to this fella and push him back if he did it again. Not ones for condoning violence ordinarily, we realised that this was to be the only real solution for Craig. He needed to stand up to this chap.

It wasn't until many months later that Craig confided in me what had happened with that situation. Barbara and I had noticed over those months that Craig hadn't come in crying. We knew something had changed but we didn't want to probe. If Craig was happy and getting on with everyone—happy days! So, months later I was standing out in the front garden with Craig talking about some cartoons when out on the path the offending boy walked by.

'Hiya Craig,' the boy said, as he walked past and on up the road.

'Hiya,' Craig replied, smiling and then looking back at me with a little glint in his eye. I returned his smile and yet said nothing, just happy to see things running smoothly for him. It was only after a minute or two that Craig offered up an explanation:

'Daddy,' he began, 'do you know how you and Mammy told me to stand up to that boy?'

'Yeah,' I answered, sensing a revelation on the cards.

'Well,' he continued, 'I did.'

'Good for you!' I said, hoping there was more to come. 'And everything is ok between you now?'

'Ah yeah,' Craig said, as he looked around again to see if the boy was anywhere around. 'He punched me ages ago but this time I didn't cry. I just grabbed him by the head and bashed it off a van.' He looked nervously at me, wondering whether I was going to give out to him or not.

I figured this was why he hadn't said anything up until that moment. I didn't quite know what to say at first. Inside I was thinking *Good man, you did right*, but on the other hand I was a tiny bit concerned at being seen to condone it. However, I knew Craig had merely acted upon the advice we had given him and was actually more bloody proud than anything else. *To hell with it . . .*

'Good man!' I said, watching as Craig's worried eyes thinned to frame a relieved smile. 'And was that the end of it?'

'Yep!' Craig answered, becoming more animated, 'and he's never done it since.' His expression was one of deep satisfaction, knowing now that he had done the right thing and that I was proud of him for doing it.

I felt obliged to include an addendum to this little chapter in Craig's life, however. I didn't want Craig walking away from this little life's lesson thinking that all situations were to be resolved this way, although I actually knew Craig understood fully anyway.

'Sometimes in life, Craig,' I said, 'we're just forced into a corner like you were and we have no choice but to do what you did.'

'I know,' Craig replied, like some old sage. I tried not to laugh at this.

'But it should always be the very last resort, ok?'

Craig smiled at me. He understood. He'd understood before I even opened my mouth. Every time he had come running home crying, it was precisely because he was not a violent person. It was not in his nature, so I knew Craig would be ok.

Craig had yet again resolved his own problem. He had faced up to it with courage and conviction and had overcome it. Barbara and I were so proud of him. Despite all the tears and all the hardship he had to endure to befriend these other boys and girls, he still kept going at it. This all came from within him. Never did we have to mollycoddle him or worry that he was becoming isolated or introverted. Like I said already, he made our role as parents so easy because of the inner strength he had. He was so mentally strong, so resilient. I can admire that quality in Craig all the more because I was so timid as a child by comparison. There was something of the invincible about Craig in the way he kept pushing through all the shit that sought to weigh him down. He'd simply keep moving, and always with a smile.

In the end he really won his friends over. Barbara and I smiled at each other one day as Craig and all his friends were in the sitting room watching a DVD. There among them was the boy who had given Craig such grief. He sat and spoke with Craig and, as fate would have it, was possibly the best mannered and charming of all the boys and girls who were there. If anything he was a little bit nervous, anxious about being in the house. So, as we witnessed this, it had apparently turned full circle, with Craig now at the centre of all these kids: he had won them over and done it all by himself.

Craig began school in September 2005 and his first year certainly was an interesting one. Barbara and I can remember how, just before he started school, he was a little bit anxious . . .

There May Be Trouble Ahead . . .

He didn't seem to be particularly concerned about 'fitting in' or express nervousness about making friends. No, Craig's worry was that he wouldn't be smart enough. We'd no idea where this came from, but he would become quite emotional at the prospect of not being able to keep up. We always knew Craig was a smart cookie so we had no worries at all on that front, and always reassured him that it would be fine. We think Craig had gotten it into his head that school was this big place where you had to know stuff already.

As soon as his first week was over he was a changed man. He knew by then what it was about and no longer had those concerns. He loved it. Barbara was the one to bring Craig to school each morning and she'd often tell me how he'd leave her at the gates to run on ahead and meet his classmates. It made the 'drop off' so much easier for both her and Craig.

There were, however, several occasions where I was lucky enough to bring Craig to school myself, but the one that stands out the most was the very first time I brought him on my own. I suppose I was a little anxious that Craig might want to stay with me but I couldn't have been more wrong. As he walked up along St Michael's Road, approaching the school with his little hand in mine, he was bursting with excitement. He pointed to people, telling me they were in his class, and quite often said 'Hello' to other kids as they passed. I thought it was fantastic. But then out of nowhere Craig let out a roar that, at first, startled me.

'Hiya Seamus!' he yelled, waving his hand in the air to someone in the distance.

I looked ahead to the crowd of adults and kids streaming in through the school gates, to see where the reaction would come. Just then, in the distance, I saw and heard.

'Howya Craig!' It was the lollypop man, complete with 'lollypop' in right hand, the other hand vigorously waving back to Craig. I was so pleased. I smiled at Seamus, giving him a cursory nod, and was just so bloody impressed with Craig's enthusiasm and friendliness. It was a revelation to me and I just couldn't help but smile.

'God, Craig you must know everyone!' I remember saying, as he just looked up at me and smiled that beautiful smile of his.

So Craig was clearly finding the transition very easy to make. This continued for the first couple of months and we were very happy with how things were going for him. In the New Year, however, 2006, some little changes began to creep in that we weren't happy with at all. It was Craig himself who had first told us that he had gotten in trouble in school. He was adamant it wasn't his fault but either way it sounded to us just like one of those things that occasionally happen in a busy classroom. We told him to try and avoid trouble and after a few words, let it go.

It was only when Barbara got called aside by Craig's teacher one morning that we began to get concerned. The teacher spoke to Barbara and explained that since the New Year Craig had become increasingly distracted in class, and she was concerned. She turned to Barbara and asked 'Is everything ok at home?' This horrified Barbara. She was so embarrassed to be asked such a loaded question and felt uncomfortable with the unnecessary implication. However, Barbara told her that everything was fine at home, and that she'd have a word with Craig about his apparently boisterous behaviour.

We confronted Craig later that evening and he told us that he was sorry. We told him we didn't want to hear of this happening anymore and that he was to behave himself in future. A few weeks went by and all was going fine. We heard nothing from the teacher, which was a good thing, and everything seemed to be back in order. But then, while in work one day, I received a call from Barbara. She told me that she had just received a call from Craig's Montessori. They had just collected Craig from school, as normal, but were informed by the teacher that we (his parents) needed to call the Principal, Sister Breda. Craig had misbehaved that day, and was apparently sent to the Principal's office.

My first reaction to this call was sheer disappointment. This was the second time that the school had sought to speak with us regarding Craig and not for the right reasons. I was eager to speak with Sister Breda as I wanted to know exactly what was going on. Craig had never been in trouble in the five years in his previous crèche, or in the current Montessori. He was such a placid boy in that respect. I wanted to get to the bottom of things and root out whatever was going wrong immediately. I didn't want this pattern continuing at all.

When I got through to the Principal she couldn't have been nicer. She just wanted a quick word to let me know that Craig had been a bit boisterous during class and that he'd spent his lunch break outside her office—just to let him know he'd done something wrong. She told me not to be worrying about him, that he was a lovely young man, and that this was just par for the course. She told me that she usually has someone outside her office each day, a tactic the school used as a deterrent for the kids. I have to say I was relieved by the light-hearted manner in which she spoke to me and by how trivial she had made the incident feel. She actually laughed as she explained how pointless Craig's experience had probably been. She said that being outside her office during lunch break was meant to be a punishment, but that when she came out to Craig he said he had a great time: there had been another boy with Craig and the two had got on exceptionally well.

I was relieved after the conversation but still wanted to put a stop to whatever was happening. I just didn't want Craig to be the one who was always getting in trouble. I knew Craig was confident and strong willed and so finding himself in trouble was probably more to do with this than anything more serious. But still, Craig should have known better and I was adamant that I was going to put an end to it. So, that evening I told Barbara that I was going to collect Craig from his Montessori, as I needed a word with him.

At about 4 p.m. I collected him. He gave me a big hug, as always, and then we headed to the car. As we drove out and away Craig chatted about this and that and all was fine. As we got a little further out the road I interrupted Craig and told him that I needed to have a very serious word with him about what happened in school. He knew instantly. Silence. I pulled the car over to a clearing just off the main road and parked up away from the edge. As I did so Craig broke the silence to rush out a hasty defence for what had happened.

'It wasn't my fault. I didn't start it!' he blurted out, panicking now and sensing he was in deep trouble.

I turned off the ignition and took off my seatbelt and turned to him. He was sitting in the front passenger seat. With a very strong and slightly raised tone I told him that his mother and I were very disappointed to be contacted by the school Principal.

'But—'

'Don't talk, Craig, just listen,' I insisted. 'You can talk when I'm finished. Ok?'

Craig just looked at me.

'Now, we're not going to move from this spot until I find out exactly what's going on,' I continued. With that Craig's expression changed. His chin wobbled and tears began to flow.

'I'm sorry, Daddy,' he cried.

'I'm sure you are sorry, Craig,' I continued, my heart going out to him as he was trapped and feeling so emotional. I wanted to reach over and give him a hug but I knew I had to nail this down. 'But I have to know what's going on here—why you are getting into trouble with your teacher so often.' I looked at him as he cried and was deadly serious . . . and he knew it. 'You're going to tell me exactly what happened today, right now, understood?'

Craig nodded.

'Off you go so!'

'This boy in my class,' Craig began, his voice warbling with the tears, 'was annoying me—it wasn't my fault,' he said.

'Tell me everything, Craig!' I interrupted. 'You didn't get in trouble because of what that boy did. You must have done something in order for the teacher to single you out. What was it?'

'He kept annoying me and calling me names and just wouldn't stop so I pushed him,' he replied, the tears still coming fast. 'The teacher called me then and I got in trouble, but it was *him* who started it.'

I believed him. I knew immediately that Craig was telling me the truth. He was right too. It wasn't really his fault at all but I knew I had to sort this. 'Ok, Craig, I can see why you were angry, but you know that you shouldn't push around like that, all right?'

'I know. I'm sorry, Daddy.'

'You're just going to have to tell your teacher when something like that happens again, ok? There's no point in you getting in trouble because of someone else. The problem for you is that the teacher doesn't see what this other boy is doing; she only sees you when you get angry or push back and that's why you're getting in trouble. And you can't push other children around like that when you're in your class, do you hear? That has to stop right now, ok?' I was firm and insistent with him. 'I believe you, Craig. I know that this other boy is the real one to blame here but he didn't get in trouble, did he?'

'No,' Craig answered, his head bent down still crying.

'So you're going to have to outsmart him and either tell your teacher when it happens again or just learn to ignore him,' I said. 'I don't want to hear about you getting in trouble again, ok?'

Craig nodded but never looked up.

'Ok, now look at me,' I continued, as his wet reddened eyes slowly peeked at me. 'You know Mammy and I love you, don't you?'

Craig nodded.

'So the first thing I want is a great big hug from you, right now.'

A shocked little smile broke on his lips, and then we reached across and gave each other a much needed bear hug. I needed it every bit as much as he did. It killed me to put him through that. The embrace was strong and Craig just let out a huge cry of 'I'm sorrrryyy, Dadddy.'

'Right. Thanks for telling me the truth, Craig,' I said as I grabbed him by the shoulders with both hands. 'Now I want to see that gorgeous smile of yours, all right?'

Craig giggled at this and looked relieved that it was all over. He moved easier in his chair and wiped the tears from his eyes.

'No more pushing, ok?'

'Yep,' he said, as he smiled a gentle little smile.

I winked at him, started the car and headed for home.

Not long after I had that roadside conversation an incident cropped up which brought everything to a head.

One night, lying on Craig's bed after making up several stories we began talking about some of the things that were on Craig's mind. I could tell there was something troubling him but I wasn't sure what. We got to chatting about school and that's when Craig looked nervously at me. He stared at me and looked like he was about to cry. 'What's wrong?' I asked.

'I'm afraid because you're going to be angry with me,' he answered, as he began to cry.

I was shocked to see him getting so upset and, holding his shoulder while he cried his heart out, I promised him that whatever it was I wouldn't get angry. He mumbled something through his tears but I couldn't hear it because he was just so emotional. I hugged him into me and just told him to relax and take his time. I was worried.

'I nearly got in trouble in school again today,' he said, crying the words out as he looked away from me. 'There's this boy in my class and he's always getting me in trouble!' he continued, the frustration and disappointment clear to see.

'What do you mean?'

'He keeps annoying me when the teacher is talking and then I get in trouble when I tell him to stop,' he said, as his teary voice changed to one of frustration. 'He's always whispering or calling my name, or sticking his pencil in me and I just get so annoyed and that's when I get in trouble. I'm always the one getting the blame and it's not my fault. I wish he'd just leave me alone.'

I knew Craig was telling the truth. He was visibly upset and frustrated at having to put up with this. He was sick of getting into trouble for things that weren't his fault. He was being provoked and it was as simple as that. As I sat there I was thinking of what I could do to help him. *I could go to see the teacher and get him to move places*, was one thought, but I just didn't want to have to bring it to that level. I started thinking and then . . .

'Maybe he fancies you?' I said, as Craig looked up at me with nostrils flared and brow furrowed.

'UUUuuughhhh, Daddy!!' he said, as he cringed at the idea.

'I tell you what, Craig; here's what you do,' I said, as Craig watched for the words. 'The next time this fella starts giving you all this attention, just turn to him and ask him does he fancy you.' I tried to show Craig just *how* he was to say it too. I told him to be really calm and demonstrated what I meant. 'Just quite calmly say "Are you gay . . . d'ye fancy me or something . . . is that why you keep trying to get my attention?" and I bet you anything he'll stop.'

I explained to Craig there are always ways to solve his problems by using his mind. I told him that the greatest thing, the most powerful thing he had was his mind and pointed to the side of his head. I stressed to him how important it was to be calm when speaking to this other boy. I said that anyone who can stay calm is really showing just how powerful their mind is. I told him that it doesn't matter how big and strong you are—if you have a powerful mind you are the real King.

Craig was very excited with this line of conversation. We sat on the bed rehearsing the conversation that he would have with this boy, with me obviously playing the part of the 'boy'. We did it over and over until Craig had his calmness and wording to a 'T'. It was great to see how empowered and joyful Craig had become in that moment. He had another option . . . and he was looking forward to using it.

A few days went by and I'd actually clean forgotten about the chat we had that night. It completely escaped my mind until I came home from work and met up with Craig. He was so excited to see me, shouting 'it worked! . . . it worked!'

'That boy started annoying me again,' Craig began, 'but this time I did what we had practised. I just turned to him and said—"Are you gay . . . do you fancy me?" I stayed really calm too.'

Craig then showed me his 'calm face' as he re-enacted the scene that had unfolded that day—word for word.

'It worked,' he said. 'He just said "Nooooo!" and looked really embarrassed and then just turned away. He didn't bother me like that anymore and I didn't get into trouble.'

'Good man, Craig,' I said, as I picked him up and showed him just how proud I was of him. And boy was I. I was so happy for him. I knew that this was such an important lesson that he'd learned. I was impressed (but not surprised) that he had seen it through and that it had worked for him. He always had been such a strong-willed little fella.

———

Before we knew it, the warm sunnier days crept in and it meant that I was home early enough for us all to go to the beach and make the most of it. Returning from the beach we'd hit the back garden and have ourselves a tasty BBQ and a beer or two. Beaches and BBQs were seemingly part of our new life and it sure did feel good. One of those afternoons at the beach proved more memorable than the rest, however . . .

Splash

It was midweek and after coming home from work we all hopped into the car and made for Ballymoney beach. This day wasn't exactly the sunniest, but it was sufficiently bright and warm to entice us along. When we got there, it was a little bit overcast, with the sun only breaking the clouds intermittently. We parked ourselves up near the shoreline and sat on the blankets and towels we'd brought along. Looking out to sea, Barbara and Craig decided they weren't swimming—the water looked too cold and unwelcoming under the greying skies. This didn't put me off, though. Within minutes I'd togged out and was in.

The water was lovely and with not a single soul in the water I had the entire shoreline to myself. I began to swim parallel to the beach, back and forth, occasionally looking back to where Barbara and Craig were based and making sure the tide wasn't sweeping me off too far. I spent a while at this, until at one point as I raised my head out of the water I thought I saw something flash past me. I stopped immediately to look around but could see nothing. *Light on the water surely.*

Thinking no more of it I resumed my swim until I reached the point where I was back in line with Barbara and Craig. Floating, I scanned the area and could see nobody else on the beach with us. The day had taken on a very grey look indeed and were it not slightly warm my being in the water would have looked like the act of a madman. It was not exactly a summer's day after all.

As I contemplated this I looked to my left, considering maybe one more swim up and down before getting out. But that's when I saw it. In my periphery I could see something black just a metre or two from me. My heart raced as I turned rapidly to see what it was. But when I actually saw what was there so close to me—almost within reach—I was gripped with fear. Two black eyes staring at me. I paused, taking in the sight before me. A large black head, long whiskers and the blackest eyes you could imagine floating within arms reach. It just stared at me. It was a seal and as I looked at its head I imagined its huge body masked beneath the water, its limbs flailing about— possibly near my stomach. I'd never felt so vulnerable in my life. I was in his domain. The thought occurred to me that maybe it was actually a mother seal whose pups were nearby and my presence in the water represented some kind of threat. Maybe she'd submerge any second and ram me in the gut, winding me, pulling me and drowning me— only metres from the shore and in view of my family.

That thought was enough. I turned instantly and thrashed the water as I headed for shore. My limbs were weak, my mind betraying me visualising the seal in submerged pursuit and about to bite off my toes. I heard Barbara from the shore saying, 'Look Craig! Look at the seal!' and then heard Craig laughing (at my display). I thrashed and flailed until finally I reached shallower water. My body felt so heavy as I clambered through the waist-high water—still not safe. I fell as the water became shallower still and my weight, weakness and terror conspired against me.

The first thing I saw was Craig's face grinning at me. He looked at my glistening flab jiggling to the fear that forced me out. I looked at him and then began to laugh. Relief, hysteria I don't know: both probably. I was safe. That was all I knew. Craig looked at me and then out to the seal who was still perched in the same spot and looking out at us (at me!). As I gasped for breath, feeling thoroughly humiliated for being so terrified of a seal, I could still see Craig looking at me.

'They can be dangerous,' I said, exhausted and pointing to the seal who from the beach perspective looked disgustingly friendly—like a cuddly toy in fact. I was trying to salvage some pride from all this but standing there wet, fat and knackered it was an impossibility. I could almost hear Craig thinking *Which one's the seal?* In the end he just looked at me, laughed and shaking his head looked back at the seal— Craig 1 Daddy 0.

Craig himself was a terrific little swimmer. He had swimming lessons every Saturday in the Forest Park Leisure Centre and he loved them. He even earned a swimming certificate for his efforts. On one of those Saturday mornings, in May 2006, I was sitting on my own in the viewing room as Craig swam happily away with his friends. Barbara was away at the time so I had brought a book with me to while away the time between winks and acknowledgements to Craig on the other side of the viewing glass. As I sat there with my coffee, reading and looking into Craig's happy energy, I had the greatest feeling of satisfaction that I can ever remember. I was thinking how lucky I was: sitting there on a bright Saturday morning enjoying a book and having a coffee while my son was happy and healthy in front of me and I with a new job that gave us so much more time with him. It was such an unfamiliar feeling and one that I welcomed deeply. It was a feeling that everything in my life had come together, at last!

LOSING...

Chapter 5

When Everything Changed

Monday, 26 June 2006 is a date I can never forget. It is the day that turned my, Barbara's and Craig's world upside down and filled my being with a fear that I didn't think could exist. In the time it takes a single moment to come and go, I went from being a strong and positive person to a trembling wreck of a man. That day began a journey whose terrible, inevitable end was marked by the cold lifeless body of our beautiful little Craig being held desperately and longingly in our arms. It was a journey we had never anticipated; a journey that dragged our hearts and souls through so much pain that we are marked forever by its unhealing wound.

This journey really began, I suppose, the day before. Barbara and I had recently noticed that Craig seemed to walk with his head slightly facing to one side. When he'd watch TV he'd seemingly stare diagonally, looking out through the side of his eyes, as opposed to watching face forward as would be normal. This had been very subtle over the previous days, but on this particular Sunday it was different. I was on my own at home watching a World Cup match on the TV while Barbara had brought Craig out to play in a local park. Sitting there, the front door opened and Barbara came quickly into the room. She was hyper and clearly anxious. She told me that we needed to bring Craig to Casualty straight away, that she knew something was seriously wrong with him.

She explained how she'd been sitting in the car while Craig had been playing on the various swings and slides, when suddenly two women had knocked on the car door window. She spoke to the ladies who told her that Craig was crying and in great distress on one of the seats. Barbara then quickly ran over and helped him out of it. He had been seated into a 'cup-like' apparatus and hadn't been able to get himself out. He had become dizzy and couldn't raise his head. Craig had been clearly upset and scared by the experience. This incident had confirmed to Barbara that something was deeply wrong and that Craig needed to get checked out.

To my eternal shame I thought Barbara was overreacting and argued that there was no need to head up to Dublin so late on a Sunday evening. I wanted to leave it till the following morning. Barbara became instantly hysterical, shouting that we had to go straight away. I swear it was only the genuine fear, determination and general hysteria I could see in Barbara that stopped me in my tracks and persuaded me to go.

While we were having this discussion in the sitting room, Craig had already run up the road to his friends. I quickly locked up the house, turned off the TV, and then made my way up to get him. As I walked up the road looking to see which house he was in I eventually saw him at a distance, with his back turned to me, speaking with friends. I called to him, saying we had to go for a drive and with that he turned and ran towards me, shouting back to his friends, 'See you later, guys.' As he ran towards me, my heart sank. His head was turned to one side, pointing downwards, but with his eyes trying to look forward. His run looked awkward and heavy footed. It was only in that moment that I too was certain something was wrong with my little boy. I couldn't understand how this had happened, and so rapidly. In that moment I felt so ashamed that I had not wanted to bring him to the hospital. I just hadn't seen it though. I really hadn't noticed how affected he'd become. When I think now of that run he made towards me, it always fills me with such dreadful sorrow and personal shame. I can't get that image out of my head.

When we finally got to the Children's Hospital in Tallaght we got to see one of the A&E doctors. He did some preliminary checks and then asked Craig to walk towards him in a straight line. His initial prognosis was that Craig perhaps had some hay-fever and that this should clear up in a few days. Both Barbara and I dismissed this out of hand and told the doctor that this was in no way a case of mere hay-fever. Hay-fever couldn't explain his sideward stare, his clumsy running, his inability to climb out of a children's park apparatus. We told him that we weren't leaving the hospital until some real tests were done. With this he arranged for a second doctor to examine Craig.

Between them they decided to organise a CAT scan for Craig the following day, so we stayed the night.

They explained that Craig had possibly contracted a virus within his brain fluid and wanted to check for inflammation in the cerebral area, with a lumbar puncture perhaps being required too. This was very concerning for us, but the doctor went out of his way to explain that it was easily remedied and that Craig would be fine. During all this Craig remained in great spirits. He never complained or showed any signs of being worried or restless even though he had to contend with different doctors coming in and getting him to do a variety of co-ordination and balance tests. We didn't know what these were about or why they were being done. The doctor explained that they were just simple routine tests to check Craig's muscle action and general co-ordination. Any inflammation in the brain area can affect this, and with Craig's condition being pinned on a viral infection of the cranial fluid these tests could help to confirm the prognosis. When I think back now on those moments I'm certain that those doctors withheld their true suspicions at that time. I'm sure they didn't want to alarm us needlessly, and I can understand that. I remember feeling worried that evening, but it was a comfortable worry. I felt that whatever may or may not be wrong with Craig we were in the right place and everything would probably be fine anyway. My fears were contained within limits, it seemed.

But that fear was still strong. I watched Craig intently, looking at his cross-eyed expression and how he tilted his head to one side when he looked at me or at anyone else who spoke to him. I watched, and I watched and watched: inspecting his movements and expressions for something new. Craig on the other hand was indifferent to all of this. His only worry was that he would be left on his own in the hospital. That sorted, he was his usual upbeat self. In fact something that Craig did that day says a lot about his character:

A number of doctors had gone through the same co-ordination checks with Craig and each time he had enthusiastically gone through the motions. On the last one of these tests a male doctor came in and introduced himself to Craig and told him that he wanted to run through some 'little tests'. Anticipating the same rigmarole Craig's reaction was to shrug his shoulders humorously and sigh, 'Not agaaain?' With that he stood at the side of the hospital bed and followed the doctor's lead with a variety of now familiar push/pull tests. I remember I was standing in the corner of the room watching this and thinking, *Why so many repeat tests in such a short time and by different doctors*? I thought it odd and quite worrying. While I was thinking this the doctor was pushing Craig's left shoulder while asking Craig to resist his efforts. Then, out of nowhere, Craig extended his right arm outwards and 'tapped' the astounded doctor in the groin. My astonishment was only surpassed by my laughter as the doctor's groin retreated instinctively upward and outward whilst he uttered a 'Whoaah!' in the process. It was safe to say that he was genuinely shocked by this unplanned 'little test' from Craig, and I'm fairly certain that in all the years that the doctor had done such tests, he'd never had his own reflexes checked by the patient—and certainly not in such a manner. I remember Barbara correcting Craig for doing this; I just stood and giggled.

This is a perfect snapshot of Craig's effervescent and wonderfully adventurous spirit. Even in that dark moment of our fear and worry, it was *he* who brought comfort to *us*. Through the sheer shining brilliance of his personality he was able to light up the room and cast out those darker thoughts from those of us around him. I often think back on that moment and it makes me smile. I see his little face and the mischief that was always written across it. I drift back into that moment and feel, once more, the glow from his presence. It is curious to me, that this moment—the very beginning of our nightmare—is the one that most frequently comes to mind when I remember Craig's true personality. It is a moment that I look back on with such warmth. You see, what I witnessed that day was not a child being 'bold' or 'rude'. No. I saw a young man with a strong, distinct personality literally 'reach out' and grab life by the balls, asserting his place in it. It was a magic moment and is a treasured memory.

That night we all slept in the hospital, with Barbara staying in the room with Craig. I don't remember much of that night. I think I must have slept ok. Barbara didn't sleep all that well though. She had wanted to sleep in the bed with Craig, but after lying with him for 'too long' Craig politely asked that she 'go to her own bed' so that he could sleep. He was too hot apparently. Craig always spoke his mind. For

Barbara, the makeshift fold-out bed—although on the floor beside Craig—was a thousand miles from the warm embrace and soft breathing of her lovely son. She wanted to hold him, keep him safe and promise that everything was going to be just fine. Sleep did not come easy to her that night.

The following morning Craig was sent down for the CAT scan. We were made to feel that this was 'no big deal' by all the staff, who no doubt were trying to shield us from the more grim possibilities. It certainly worked on me. Barbara was more nervous than I was, that's for sure. I truly felt that we were just going through the motions that day: at worst a confirmation of the viral infection would be given; a course of treatment would follow and Craig would eventually return to full health in no time. I was always the optimist.

When we arrived for the scan, Craig was talked through what would happen. He was then laid out on the bed, his head secured into position with tape. The CAT scan itself was like a large polo mint with a bed through the middle. Craig was absolutely fine throughout the scan. We looked out at him from behind a glass door in a separate room. I hated seeing him out there. There's something instinctively wrong for parents to watch their child from a position of safety, while the child lies exposed and in harm's way. And even though you can reason it out in your mind, there's a part of you that wants to run in and take him up in your arms. That is how I felt. While the scan was underway Barbara became uncomfortable with the number of doctors in the room who were looking at the images generated. She turned to me and quietly said, 'That can't be good, that amount of doctors, can it?' As always I reasoned it out in some harmless way and when the scan was finally over we returned to Craig's room.

Shortly after, a nurse came to the room and told us that the doctor would be with us at 2 p.m. with the results from the scan. Grand, I thought. Barbara was still anxious but I was calm. Somewhere in my brain there seems to be a programme that prevents all 'per chance' and therefore unnecessary worry and stress—a code which only allows actual 'real-time' occurrences to bring about those pangs of fear. While we waited that morning I can honestly say that it was no different than if we were just waiting for an everyday prescription for antibiotics. I had come to fully believe that Craig had probably contracted some temporary, treatable infection and that there was no cause for serious concern: the doctor would meet us at 2 p.m., confirm the infection and then talk us through a fixed course of oral medication. This was just standard illness treatment and all would be grand in time.

When 2 p.m. arrived, there was no sign of the doctor. A few minutes later the same nurse came back into the room and told us that the doctor was on his way. Again, 'grand' I thought—we won't have to wait around all day, as can often happen in hospital situations. The nurse's word was good and within a few minutes the doctor opened the door. The nurse came into the room too and said that she would stay with Craig while we spoke to the doctor in a separate private room. This piece of information didn't fit the mould of my expectation and it was the first moment something stirred in my stomach. I knew something was wrong. Barbara looked at me, the same concern written all over her face. We turned to Craig before leaving and told him we'd only be a few minutes. When we walked out from the room and onto the corridor there were a number of doctors waiting outside, and as we walked to the 'private room' they all walked alongside us. This moment is still so vivid in my mind now. It was this moment when the protective programme and its code broke down in my head and fear began to flow uncontrollably into my mind. I looked at Barbara and I could see the same fear mirrored back. The uncomfortable and telling silence between all of us as we walked to that room—only metres away—ripped away at every shred of strength and composure that I'd relied on.

We were gestured into the room and to two seats. Then, all of a sudden, we were surrounded by the doctors and a nurse. I could feel a weakness running through my body as the oppression of that drawn-out moment became almost impossible to bear. Barbara's face told of what mine struggled to hide. We were terrified. There was no denying that we were about to be told something 'bad'. It was a female Indian doctor who eventually spoke first: 'Ok, Mr and Mrs Sexton, we've had a look at the results of your son's CAT scan and I'm sorry to say there appears to be a prominent tumour in his lower brain area . . .'

Two things happened instantly when those words were spoken: my throat froze and Barbara screamed. In an instant it was as if I was outside myself. I kept looking at the doctor, but every muscle in my body was still—numb. I could feel and hear the pulse in my neck and the gathering of doctors and nurses in the room seemed distant somehow. Barbara's screams of—'Nooo . . . Nooo . . . Is he going to die . . . Is my baby going to die?' were the only thing that kept me grounded in the room. I reached for Barbara and held her, knowing that I couldn't give any comfort, but feeling like it was *us* against *them*. The only thing louder in my head than Barbara's screaming questions was the non-committal answers in reply. What wasn't said floored me. Never had I been gripped by such utter terror in my life. The consultant paused briefly, allowing for our reaction, before continuing to discuss the results.

I watched as her mouth moved, but my mind, for a moment, wasn't capable of fully taking it all in. All I could picture was my beautiful little Craig only metres away in his room, playing and chatting with the nurse—oblivious to the evil manifestation lying within his head. In some illogical way I felt like I was betraying him—being told about his serious condition while he knew nothing of it. All I could think of was Craig saying 'See you later, guys' to his friends the day before, and wondering just how long that 'later' would be. I was devastated. Barbara was devastated and looked visibly shook. For her it was beyond her worst fears. She had known all along that something was wrong—really wrong. But never had she allowed herself to think that the death of her son was a possibility.

When all was finally said, we both left the room, making our way out to the outside corridor. In the relative privacy it provided, we hugged each other, crying uncontrollably and squeezing desperately into each other. *Our precious little boy is dying.* We were powerless in this situation. There was nothing on this earth that could make this pain go away. Nothing that could reverse what we'd just been told. Nothing that could stop this reality from being ours. We were drowning in fear and torment and there was nothing or no one that could rescue us— rescue Craig. The helplessness and the hopelessness in that moment was so powerful that it just consumed us both, completely. I was weak. Barbara was weak. Yet, we had to be the strongest we could ever be— if only to walk back into Craig's room and face our dying son with the masks that were expected of us.

Barbara decided that she wanted to ring her mother first and let her know. She, along with my own parents, already knew we had Craig in hospital and were due to come in later that day. I decided that I should

ring my parents too. When I rang them, they had me on speaker phone
in the car. When I tried to speak, I couldn't mouth the words. All that
travelled down the phone were the obvious sounds of my despair—
stifled tears and unfamiliar high-pitched exhalations. My mother tried
desperately to get some sense from me:

'Neville . . . what's wrong?'

Silence.

'Is it Craig? . . . Is he ok? . . . Tell us.'

Silence . . . Tears . . . Gurgling. My throat was frozen.

'Neville . . . Please!' said with quickly deteriorating emotion and
dread.

Tears.

'Is it Craig? . . . Is it bad, Neville?'

'Yes . . .'

It was all I could do to say that single word. I couldn't say the
horrific words that needed saying. My body wouldn't allow it. My
father then interrupted saying, 'Neville, we're on our way to the
hospital now . . . we'll see you very shortly.'

Barbara was at the other end of the corridor and was speaking on
the phone to her mother. I was still lost in a haze of disbelief as I
heard her saying words like 'Craig', 'tumour' and 'dying'—words that
stabbed me in the heart with each utterance. After the call, Barbara
told me her mother was on the way up to the hospital. We looked at
each other, composed ourselves, and agreed that we had to go back to
Craig.

I rubbed away the tears and took a number of deep sniffs to clear my
nose and throat. I asked Barbara whether my face looked ok, and
reassured her that her own was fine. We approached the door, opened
it, and entered the room.

Craig was sitting upright on the bed, talking with the nurse and
playing with something. When I looked at him I just drank him in. I
wanted to run over and hold him so tight. I wanted to be his dad and
protect him from the world. Craig looked up and smiled at us both; we
smiled back. The nurse made some polite conversation, telling us
emphatically that they'd 'had great fun' while we were gone, before
finally leaving us to be alone with our son. We walked over and sat on
his bed and, trying not to be overly tactile, gave him hugs and kisses
while asking him what he'd been doing while we were gone.

'That was longer than a few minutes,' was Craig's immediate and factual reaction. We never could bullshit Craig; he was always too cute for that.

We watched Craig intently as he spoke. We dared not look at each other. I guess we were afraid that we'd crumble if our eyes met. We spoke with him. We smiled with him. We sang with him. He sat on our knees and talked while we listened. It was such a powerful experience to watch over our child, whose future—only moments before—had been stolen. It is beyond my abilities to truly convey how we felt in that room. I guess it needs to be felt to be understood. Only parents who've suffered the same tragedy can know, I suppose.

As we sat in the room I remember struggling to keep my eyes from weeping. I couldn't let him see something was wrong. Craig was especially intuitive too, always picking up on people's emotions, so it was difficult to keep mine from him. He'd never seen me cry before. If he did, I was certain he'd know something was not right. At one point, I lay on the floor of the hospital room with my back against the wall. Craig came over and sat on my lap. His back was turned into mine. I just stared at the back of his head. I kept staring at it, asking, begging God to make it go away and leave my son alone. I held Craig tightly and kissed the top of his head. With his back turned to me, the tears just flowed from my eyes. The heat from his body, the smell of his hair— all now temporary: I was holding my beautiful dying boy.

After a while we were told that one of the doctors wanted to see us. He began by telling us that Craig would need to be moved to Crumlin Hospital to receive the specialised care required. He also wanted to speak with us because he felt we were perhaps unclear on what we'd been told and that all hope was not in fact lost, as our appearance and demeanour implied. He explained that 'many brain tumours—about ninety per cent in fact—are entirely operable, with the child returning to full health once the tumour is removed.'

When I heard this I felt hope returning. I had certainly left the previous consultation feeling that we'd been told that Craig was going to die. But this doctor had offered us a lifeline. I sat wide-eyed looking at him, a new energy coursing through my veins. The dark mist in my mind had shifted. *Craig could make it after all.* When we left the room I kept repeating what the doctor had said. We both felt terrified but now there was room for optimism—for hope. We hugged each other before returning to Craig.

Shortly after that our families began to arrive. We were in the room with Craig when the door opened slightly. The nurse popped in to tell us that we had visitors and that she would sit with Craig while we went outside to speak with them. It was my mother and father, along with Barbara's mother, Breda, and sister Shirley. We stepped outside the room, leaving the nurse with Craig, and the emotions just burst out. Neither Barbara nor I could hold back the tears and the terror that had been welling up inside us. All I can remember is walking down to the end of that corridor and telling them, through tears and a crumbling voice, that our precious Craig had a brain tumour. Up until that point my parents hadn't got a clue what to expect. Somehow saying the words out loud terrorised me to the core. It made it even more real. I remember the shocked expression on my mother's face and how my father just shook his head. Barbara was a bit further down, speaking with Breda and Shirley. I could see and hear the tears coming from where she stood.

Breda came up to meet us then and gave me a hug, trying to console me. I was a wreck. Barbara was destroyed. She told me to go back down to Barbara. Our life was in complete tatters. The hope that we had, from hearing that most tumours were operable, seemed gone at that moment. The terrifying reality that they were going to have to open Craig's skull and start slicing at his brain filled us with nothing but fear. I recall, however, after the initial revelation how I seemed to calm slightly. I started to cling desperately to that hope once more. *It's just like another operation*, we started to tell ourselves. *Craig will go asleep and wake up ok. Maybe a little scarred, but alive!* This is what we grabbed onto and couldn't let go. Within us both, this hope was all that we focused on.

Craig was delighted with the visitors. He was in great form. From his excitement you'd never have known there was a gun pointed at his head. He carried on regardless, delighted by all the attention and the audience for his singing. He sat on his bed singing song after song and smiled that beautiful smile of his through every word and note. But for us around him, there was such beauty and such tragedy in what we watched. Barbara and I smiled and laughed with him as he belted out those songs but I could see in Barbara, and she in me, the devastation that lay concealed. We could see the gun.

Later that evening Barbara and I were called to see one of the doctors again. This was never good news and we were scared. We were brought to the specialist's room and he sat us down to explain Craig's condition in more detail. He wanted to be as honest as he could be and began telling us what he knew. He told us that the particular tumour that Craig had was in his brain stem and that he believed it was inoperable. This knocked us: the hope we'd been given was at once taken away. I desperately started quizzing him about malignancy and benignity but he was quick to point out that this was most likely irrelevant. He told us that a biopsy would be needed to determine malignancy but that this was not an option in Craig's case, because of the tumour location. Blow after blow rained down on us in that room and we simply couldn't take any more. 'You're telling us that there's no hope for Craig then?' is all I could muster, looking at the doctor through blurred vision. We were defeated by his uncompromising honesty.

'There's always hope,' is all he could say. But that honest answer felt equally damning. For a specialist consultant with years of training and experience to only offer us 'hope' was the final blow. I just nodded my head and looked at the ground and then Barbara. *Medicine could not save our boy.* He finished by saying that we'd have to wait until the specialist oncologists from Crumlin Hospital gave their opinion. They were the real experts, he said.

We walked out of that room slowly, and with a weakness that only such news can bring. Nurses laughed somewhere down the corridor while our little boy lay dying in another room and while we stood as two ruined people just outside. We came back quietly into Craig's room and relieved the nurse who was by now good friends with Craig. We sat with him and talked and buried our own nightmarish thoughts. We couldn't let him know what we knew. My stomach churned and squirmed with the heavy truth that it could not ignore. I also felt like such a traitor, holding back the truth from Craig. We both did. We sat in that room playing and smiling alongside him and we kept the devastating truth far away from him. But how could we possibly tell him that he was so sick. It would have been so unfair to burden him with it. He would have been scared and so alone. We couldn't do it.

As I hugged Craig on the bed I became incensed with anger and frustration. I was so angry that the other doctor had given us such false hope. He clearly knew nothing of Craig's condition and should never have been allowed to misadvise so. I even allowed for the fact that he was only trying to help us and that his advice came from some noble place, born from a caring heart. I allowed for all this but my anger at being so blatantly misled, about something so life-changing, burned in me. I began to question the doctors' expertise then. I questioned how one doctor could say one thing, and another something so different—so damning. I questioned whether Craig was in the best place, whether the best minds were looking at his condition. I immediately requested a meeting with the specialist to discuss all this. There was no time to waste and I wanted to know the truth about everything.

I sat down with the specialist and told him that I would do *anything* to give Craig the best chance he could have. I made it very clear that we would stop at nothing to get Craig the best treatment there is. Barbara and I would sell our house and raise whatever money was needed if it meant Craig could have a better chance anywhere else in the world. Beforehand, my father made it absolutely clear that they would do the same. We urgently needed for this doctor to understand that money was not in any way a concern when it came to Craig's situation. I didn't want him withholding options for Craig out of some inaccurate belief that we may not be in a position to finance it. This was paramount for me to get across to the doctor.

Jesus Christ, there was no way we would allow something as transient and unreal as money to ever come between our Craig and his life. If we had no money we would find it. I expressed this very clearly to the doctor and made it equally clear that if there was a better place on this planet to help Craig then I needed to know where it was. In fairness to the doctor he listened to what I had to say and both recognised and understood the unfaltering desperation with which I engaged him. But he told me straight. If Craig's tumour was the particular beast that he believed it to be—and he was careful to remind me that it needed to be confirmed by the specialists in Crumlin Hospital first—then the tragedy was that it was simply an inoperable one. He told me that there was no hospital or clinic in the world that offered anything superior to what we had in this country for conditions such as Craig. He assured me that Crumlin Hospital would offer Craig the best of what is currently available and that carting Craig to the other side of the world was neither advisable nor necessary.

My head dropped. I had lost control over the situation again. I really thought that there was hope to be had elsewhere in the world—America perhaps—but no. Any sense of being able to resolve this nightmare kept slipping away. There was nothing we or anyone could do for Craig and it was fucking killing us. I wanted to scream at how this could be happening to us, to Craig. *Why, why, why hadn't medicine improved in treating cancer? This can't be true! This can't be bloody happening! Not our Craig . . . Not our beautiful precious Craig . . . For fuck's sake why won't someone help us! We can't just let him die . . .*

I returned to the room and took Barbara outside to tell her the news. The emptiness and the rawness that we both felt is indescribable. All we could do was go back into the room with Craig and spend time with him. We were so lost and the pain of sitting there looking at him was just so impossible to bear. He was everything to us. Everything. This situation was so unspeakably horrific that it was almost inconceivable for us to accept. But no matter what we did, thought or said, there it was—the truth. Craig is dying. It took over our minds and shadowed our every thought. Death was with us and it placed its stenching mouth over ours, denying us a breath—smothering us.

Later that night I returned to the parent's spare room which I'd been staying in. Sleep was not on my mind. I was tired, so very tired, but my mind was filled with a thousand fears. I felt so powerless. I lay on the bed, outside the covers in my clothes, and just cried my heart out. I cried like a baby. I roared and wailed in the solitude of that room as I finally allowed the torrent of fears to wash over me. I cried and I cried and I still kept crying. There was no end to this pain that took over my body. All that kept going over and over in my mind was that Craig was going to die. He was never going to grow up. We had always looked after him. We'd been by his side in everything he did. Every new experience he had we were there to hold his hand. But in dying he would walk alone. He would be scared and his mammy and daddy would not be there to hold his hand. This filled me with such terror that I remember my hands shaking in the bed. The thought 'I'm his daddy, it's my job to protect him, and I'm going to let him down,' kept reeling through my head. 'I love him so much and I can't help him. He's going to die and not have his mammy or daddy to comfort him.' My mind haunted me all night.

But then something occurred to me, something I hadn't thought of before, and a calmness washed over me. I stopped crying. I stopped shaking. I felt something akin to peace. As I was lying there with the tumult of a thousand fears strangling and scratching my mind, the thought 'We'll go with him' suddenly jumped to the fore. With all sincerity and with one hundred percent conviction I held onto this thought and knew that I would do it. I almost felt excited by the awakening within me that I had a choice in this. I was not powerless. Before this thing could take Craig, before he suffered at all, we could go together as a family. I lay there and visualised how it would be done. I saw us walking into our garage, with Craig asleep in my arms and all of us sitting into the car. We would take some sleeping pills perhaps and just before I'd fall asleep I'd start the car. I would leave the windows down and we'd wake up together in the afterlife. It seemed peaceful and perfect. We would not be parted. We would be together—as a family should be. Craig would not be abandoned to face this journey alone. I thought this through and then quietly, serenely fell asleep.

In the morning I awoke to the nightmare once more. I started the day with the heaviness of the very real terror that now cloaked me. But in the back of my mind was this 'way out'. It comforted me to know that if the worst came we'd be with Craig all the way. We had control again. I quickly got dressed and made my way to Craig's room. Craig was full of energy but Barbara looked terrible. She hadn't slept at all. She'd been smothering her tears all night and did not want Craig to hear her. I hugged Craig hard into me and gave him a loving kiss. He looked at me strangely but I just smiled at him. Barbara went for her shower first. There was a shower room just up the corridor and she wasn't long. I played with Craig and we talked. The nurse—Craig's friend—then came in to the room and offered to mind Craig while I went for a shower. While sharing the room with Barbara and watching her fall apart with uncontrollable tears I decided to tell her what I had thought of. I told her that we had another option: I explained that we could go with him. But when Barbara heard this, she just looked at me. She was absolutely shocked at what I'd come out with.

'I can't believe you said that!' she said. 'You would commit suicide!'

Hearing Barbara say it back to me like that made me feel ridiculous. I looked at her and told her that it was just something that I had thought of during the night. I even explained how we could do it. But the more I spoke the more perplexed and disturbed Barbara looked. 'Are you fucking serious?' she asked, and all I could do was say I dunno.

I quickly distanced myself from the idea, however, seeing how much it troubled Barbara. It obviously was something that she could never consider. I rubbished the idea and then changed the subject.

––––

That day Craig had a number of visitors. Marie Kennedy—who in her crèche in Bray had looked after Craig from the time he was just a 3-month-old baby right up to the age of five—came to visit that afternoon. She met us outside and shared tears in the corridor. Craig loved Marie dearly and Marie loved him like a son. They were a team, having spent all those long days in the crèche together as he grew up. Craig was always the first to arrive in the mornings and quite often the last to leave too. I simply cannot overstate how important Marie was in Craig's life. But she and Craig hadn't seen each other in nearly a year at that point and Marie was devastated to hear of his tumour.

Craig was so happy to see her. They gave each other a big hug and Craig's face lit up like a light. She had brought him a wonderful gift. It was a mug with a superimposed photo of her and Craig from their time in the crèche together. 'Oh wow!' Craig said, followed by, 'Thank you, Marie.' He loved it. Marie eventually left and asked us to keep in touch. She gave Craig another big hug before turning and walking out of the room.

Later that evening a gentleman came to the room and had with him a piece of cloth from the glove of Padre Pio. My Aunt Marie had contacted him and asked him to come to see Craig. He came in to the room and said hello to Craig and told him that he was going to say a nice little prayer for us all. I've never been a religious man, nor was Barbara, but there was nothing that we wouldn't try to help Craig. When he was ready we all stood around Craig who was still sitting up in his bed. The man began reciting a Hail Mary and we all followed suit. As we came to the end of the prayer, Craig, to the background of our silence, began speaking confidently and loudly all on his own—'St Brigid of Ireland help us; we pray for your love and your guidance . . .' We all just stopped and listened. We looked down and watched as he smiled his way through a prayer that I'd never heard of before. I was startled, but so very proud of how our little Craig just asserted his prayer so confidently while surrounded by so many. It never phased him. After each Hail Mary he repeated his prayer, to all our adoring smiles and glistening eyes. It was a beautiful moment and yet another example of Craig's capacity to surprise us. He was such a special soul.

The next day we were scheduled to be moved to Crumlin Hospital, where Craig's treatment plan would begin. We were so desperate to hear what the experts in Crumlin had to say about Craig's scans. We had already been told the worst, so we were left with only the hope for something more. Barbara and I were completely overwhelmed by the brick wall of negativity and total surrender by those in Tallaght. I had asked my brother Darren, who himself is a PhD and lecturer in Immunology in UEA, to find out what he could through any contacts he might have. He rang me back not long after and pretty much confirmed what the specialist had told me. However, he also mentioned a place in the States—Colorado University—which would be worth contacting, just for a second opinion. This place was a world leader in such treatments and so their opinion would be vital for us. We instantly jumped at this chance, and embraced the hope that it gave. But first we needed to hear what Crumlin had to say.

The next morning a taxi was arranged to bring us to Crumlin Children's Hospital. On the way, the nurse who travelled with us asked whether we had been to St John's ward in Crumlin before. This is where Craig would be staying. We told her we hadn't and she instantly felt obliged to warn us of what we'd see. She explained that there were a lot of very sick children there and that they were quite visibly so. She also explained that the ward was an old one and that it would be a very different experience to that in Tallaght Hospital. She felt we needed to know this before arriving. Barbara and I looked at each other and felt a sinking sensation within. However, we were too focused on the meeting with the oncologist to really absorb or take heed of what the nurse had said. Craig's health was the only thing that mattered to us.

As we entered St John's ward it was immediately evident that it was worlds apart from where we'd just been. The first thing to hit us was the heat. It was incredibly warm and there seemed to be an element of chaos as we progressed down the ward. There was a radio playing loudly somewhere and it filled the air. As we passed different rooms, TVs and videos seemed to scream out a multitude of competing programmes, none of which could be discerned through the mix of noise. Children looked out from the rooms with sunken eyes and hairless heads. A beautiful little girl, just skin and bone, was wheeled past us and her sad little eyes looked up at us as she braved a smiling hello. Her arms were so thin. My heart was broken. I hugged Craig closer to me and fought the urge to run out the door and keep Craig from all this. We worried what was going through Craig's mind as he passed along. *What must he be thinking?*

Standing in the corridor, it felt as if nobody was expecting us. We seemed to be waiting around for ages before eventually being told that there was no bed. We were led into a room with two beds and a cot. We had to put Craig into the cot because there simply wasn't a bed for him. I looked at Craig as he sat there, humiliated and so despondent with being treated like a baby. 'It's not fair,' he said. He was so right. Barbara and I looked around in horror at what was all about us. We sat there, with Craig in the cot looking miserable, and with two TVs in the room all facing away from Craig and playing some loud toddler videos. We were trapped in this nightmare. There was no dignity in it. All the windows were closed, to limit infections, but leaving the place feeling so uncomfortably hot. There was just heat and noise everywhere and we were so angry—so scared. We had to wait there until the specialist did his rounds and nobody could give us a time as to when that would be.

We took Craig out of the room because it was just too oppressive and brought him down to where we were told the playroom was. When we walked in I was disgusted. The place was like some abandoned storage room. There were bits and pieces of broken toys everywhere and the fact that there were no children there when we arrived, spoke volumes. We hid our disgust from Craig and tried to keep positive for him. We found some air hockey table (with no air) and tried playing a game. If anything, the relative peace in this room gave us some space to breathe, so we stayed for as long as we could. But there was no denying the grim reality of the place where we now were.

It was horrendous and so unfair to the children there. These were the sickest children in the country and they were all tucked away in some shithole ancient corridor with no privacy, comfort or dignity, or even a lousy working toy to play with. It was an absolute scandal. These children deserved so much more. It was absolutely inexcusable for these beautiful, delicate little kids to have to endure this horrendous environment. I was so appalled to see the reality of this situation first-hand. I couldn't understand how this could be. All my life I'd seen fundraising events and collections for Crumlin; every small town and village seemed permanently engaged in such collections. *So where the hell was all the money going?* I thought. It appeared that these poor unfortunate children were of least importance to those who controlled the purse strings.

The other thing was that we were told that we couldn't bring Craig out from the ward—something he desperately wanted to do. We wanted to take him out to get some food in the canteen but we couldn't. We were told that Craig had to stay there at all times for hygiene purposes. But even that was ludicrous. People were walking in and out of the ward all day so there was no logic in the imposed limitation in terms of health risk. Craig coming and going was no different than Barbara or I or other visitors, and him leaving posed no extra risk to himself or the other children. If the limitation was imposed for the sake of contactibility this could have been worked around in any number of ways. There was no sense in Craig being confined like that and he really could have done with getting away, if only for a short while.

We were so angry and couldn't bury the feeling that we weren't doing our best by Craig. We sat there and looked around, feeling helpless, but at all times trying our best not to let Craig see it. But Craig already had his own mind made up. While sitting in the cot and after absorbing his surroundings he turned to his mammy and just cried. 'Please, Mammy, don't let me stay here,' he begged. It was the first time I'd seen Craig so visibly distressed and depressed by the situation. Our hearts bled for him. I had a lump in my throat and I came so close to just picking him up, walking out the door and away from this torment. But I couldn't. We told him that we would do everything to get us all home, but that if we had to stay we'd all stay together.

Finally, after a long wait, we got to see the oncologist—but not in private. The oncologist just came into the shared room and pulled across the thin curtain to speak with us. Before he said a word, we could hear the two TVs in the room being turned down and the up-until-then incessant conversation grew silent. As the oncologist spoke it was for everyone in that room to hear. It was terrible.

He confirmed that Craig's tumour was the nastiest one and that it was inoperable. He told us that it was terminal and that it was really only a matter of time. The best he could tell us was that in the ten or so years of children in Crumlin with this tumour, there was only one girl who still lived. Like Craig, she developed the tumour when she was five and was now ten years old and still living. But even with that, the oncologist told us, her tumour was a time-bomb. We were left destroyed. He looked down upon us with that necessarily thick-skinned medical sympathy, which no doubt disappeared as soon as he walked out the door, and when we had no further questions, left us be.

We cried behind those curtains and knew that those strangers on the other side had heard it all. But that didn't matter. All that mattered was that our son had been given a definitive death sentence and there was nothing on earth now that could be done. The pain was too much.

We knew we had to meet with another consultant, Dr O'Meara, to get more information, and so with Craig, Shirley and Breda we headed to the new consultants' wing for our appointment. It's amazing really, but as we entered this brand new modern block with its beautiful fountain and serene atmosphere, it was Craig who first said what we were all thinking—'How come this place is so nice and where I am is so horrible?' He was right. This multimillion plush consultants' wing screamed out at us. Why in hell something so extensive and costly was allowed to be built for consultants when there were so many horrifically sick children living in terrible conditions only metres away, was beyond me. I was incensed by the insensitivity of it. The fact that Craig had immediately felt it was the real measure of how hurtful its grotesque splendour was. There was no justification for it. If I was a consultant, I thought, I simply could not in all conscience sit there, knowing the truth of what lay on the other side of the hospital.

But incensed as I was, as we all were, it was very much at the back of my mind. Shirley and Breda stayed with Craig as we headed in to see Dr O'Meara. We sat down and listened as she explained Craig's condition to us yet again. But then she gave a most horrible answer to Barbara's surprising question: 'How long has he got?'

'Seven to nine months.'

That was it, my resistance was gone. My mind froze. My heart froze. Barbara just wept; my eyes surrendered to the tears. We held each other as the fear coursed through our veins. It was too much to take. It's hard for me to get across the state of my mind, and Barbara's, in that moment. This was the culmination of all our deepest fears in life. Blow after blow after blow had hit us since we first took Craig up to Tallaght Hospital and with each delivery we were beaten back down to the floor. But those horrible words finished it. All hope was lost and our poor little boy, sitting innocently outside in the corridor, was unaware that his life—his death—had been fixed. He had months only. *Months?*

We sat together in that room, lost in our own thoughts, and listened as Dr O'Meara repeated her words of 'sorry' to us both. There was nothing in the world that could make this go away. Nothing. Dr O'Meara began to speak about Craig's treatment plan and how we were to progress over the next few months, and although I knew I had to listen all I could see was Craig in my mind. I could see him outside sitting on the chair talking away with enthusiasm and joy and just so full of life. *Full of life?*

Just then a second oncologist came in to the office and without any warning produced a scan of Craig's brain, pointing out to us the area and size of the tumour. She matter-of-factly told us that it was the size of an egg and that in time Craig would begin a degenerative cycle with the loss of muscle use, eventually culminating in his inability to swallow and ultimately in his death. It was like an avalanche. It was so unspeakably horrific to sit there and be confronted with this night-mare truth. Knowing Craig was to die was harrowing beyond words, but to then understand that he was going to suffer in death made us weak and sick to our bones. Our sweet, innocent, beautiful Craig did not deserve this. This was gruesome and barbaric and beyond comprehension.

Neither Barbara nor I could speak at that moment. I think we both wanted to lie down, curl into a ball and never wake up. How could we face Craig now? How could we allow this to happen to him? We stood there in the room, saying nothing, as both doctors looked at us. The door opened and a colleague stuck her head in to say what time they were all 'going to lunch at'. Dr O'Meara apologised to us for this, but no matter. We stood, but inside we were on our knees. Everything was lost. There was nothing of hope left to us and all we now had was fear.

We both looked at each other knowing that it was time to go and that we had to hide our pain from Craig. We braced ourselves and walked out the door. Down the corridor and through a glass door partition we could see him sitting with Breda and Shirley. He looked around and stared right at us. We could see his smile and his excitement and we walked silently towards him. We came through the door and gave him a big hug and a kiss before grabbing his little hand to begin walking away. Breda and Shirley looked at us both and they knew.

When we got back to the ward Shirley took Craig aside, allowing Barbara to confide in her mother. Barbara sobbed bitterly as she explained what we'd been told. It was truly the stuff of nightmares. I remember meeting my mother when she came in and breaking down as I told her the news. I cried like a child. I buried my head in my hands and erupted into an uncontrollable fit of tears. I was shaking with the emotion that took control of me. My father came down the corridor just moments later and was utterly devastated by the news. I stood there crying my heart out and thought of how hard Craig's life had been. I was overcome with despair and regret; regret at how we'd never done enough for him. How we'd both worked which resulted in Craig spending most of his life in a crèche. How he never got all the birthday parties that he wanted. I was so angry and so hopelessly lost that I could barely breathe. I felt responsible in all this and couldn't escape the torment that I had failed Craig as a father. He was only a little boy and not meant to suffer like this. I was meant to keep all that away and protect him until he was grown up. But instead I was standing by while all this was happening to him. I pictured him looking up at me with fear in his eyes while I stood powerless to help him. It burned in my stomach and I cried for it not to be.

———

Preparations for Craig's treatments began very soon after this. He required that a plastic mask be moulded perfectly to his face which was then precisely marked for the radiotherapy. This was no simple task and I'm not speaking about the expertise required. I'm talking about what Craig had to endure. He had to lie flat on a bed as a heated, softened lattice of plastic was pushed over his face and into the contours of his head. The plastic was necessarily hot and Craig was required to remain perfectly still as it was pushed and moulded into the very shape of his head and face. Standing there I could feel a claustrophobic feeling coming over me. Watching, I was in complete admiration as he struggled through and braved the ordeal. For most people, under normal circumstances, this would be a very uncomfortable and difficult experience to have to go through, but for Craig the situation was much more complicated.

You see one of the big obstacles for Craig prior to this, the one that scared him most, was the dizziness he felt as he lay flat on his back. Yet another cruel side effect of the tumour, Craig's balance would often be shot as he lay back into a horizontal position. He would panic, struggle and cry as his head began to lower. As he approached the horizontal position he would hyperventilate through tears and pull himself backwards in a reactive instinct to stop the dizzy nauseating feeling that was hitting him. So Craig had to first fight through this disorientation—mentally overcome it—before then suffering the additional smothering sensation of the hot mask. I don't know how he did it, but he did. There were tears—of fear and anger—but still he persisted doggedly until it was done.

Once the mask was fitted properly, Craig had to get up and move to another room and further endure another long, arduous process. This time he had to lie down on a table (overcome the nausea and disorientation again) and remain perfectly still for almost forty minutes while various lasers were used to position and mark out points on the mask. To ensure that the mask and Craig's head remained still, the bottom of the mask was secured with blocks to the bed. This fixed his head stock still; again a very uncomfortable experience. But Craig got through it.

Once all this was complete, Craig was finally ready to begin his course of radiotherapy treatment out in St Luke's Hospital. It was a frightening enough prospect for us his parents, let alone for Craig who had to go through it. Prior to that first week of treatment we had been told that we could bring a CD player into the room so that Craig could listen to whatever he wanted while the treatment was going on. So, I remember how on his first day we did exactly that.

That first treatment was memorable for a whole number of reasons but the one nice memory that stands out involved the words of a stranger. Craig had been in having his treatment while an elderly man was outside waiting for his turn. Craig had brought his CD player into

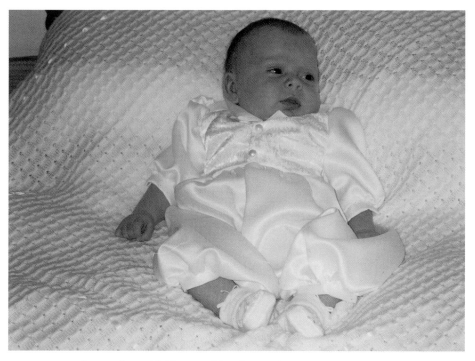

Ever so proud—our beautiful boy on his Christening Day (2000).

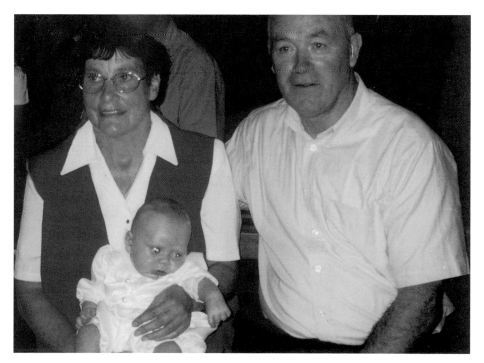

Craig with his Nana and Granddad Sinnott (Christening Day, 2000).

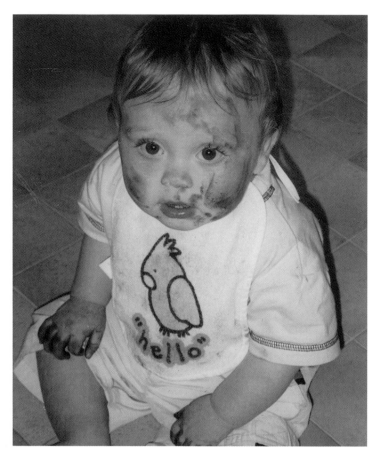

Craig, after finding what was in the coal bucket! (2001).

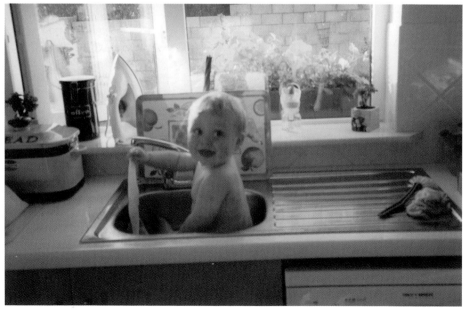

'Emergency wash' after Craig had found the coal bucket (2001).

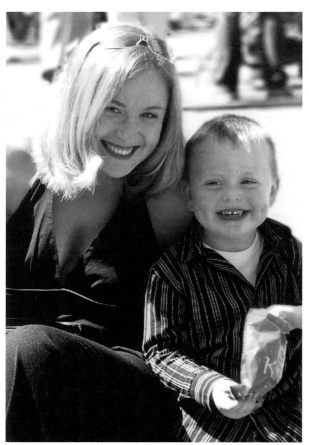

Craig with his aunty Mel—
a lovely photo of our
beautiful boy.

Our little family with
Craig, aged three.

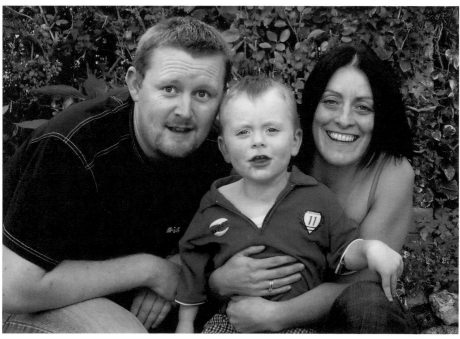

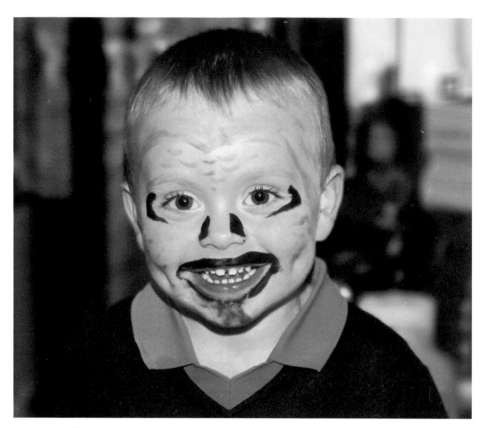

Our beautiful, happy Craig, aged three.

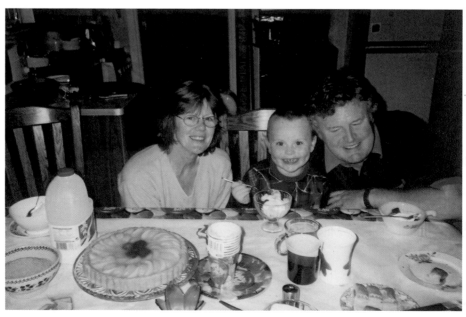

Craig with his Nana and Granddad Sexton (2004).

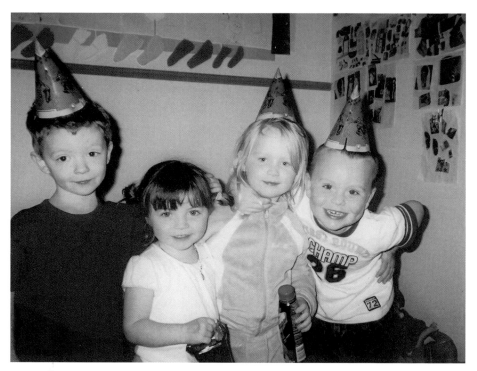

Craig celebrating with his crèche buddies in Bambinos, Bray (2004).

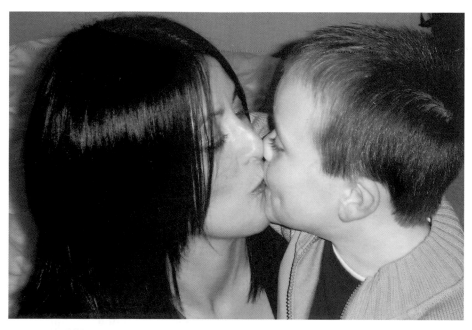

A treasured kiss, a moment captured—Mammy and Craig (2005).

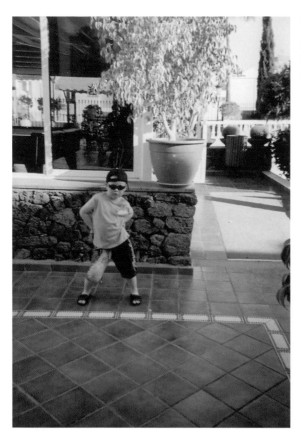

'Mr Cool Dude'—Craig posing outside the apartment while on holidays in Lanzarote (2005).

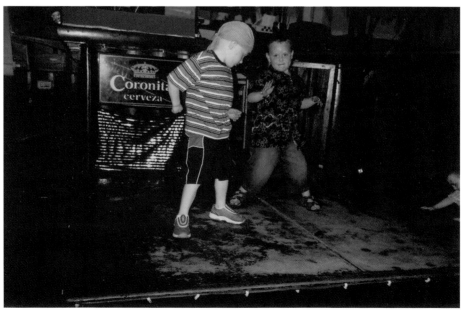

'He's the greatest dancer'—Craig busting some moves on holiday in Lanzarote (2005).

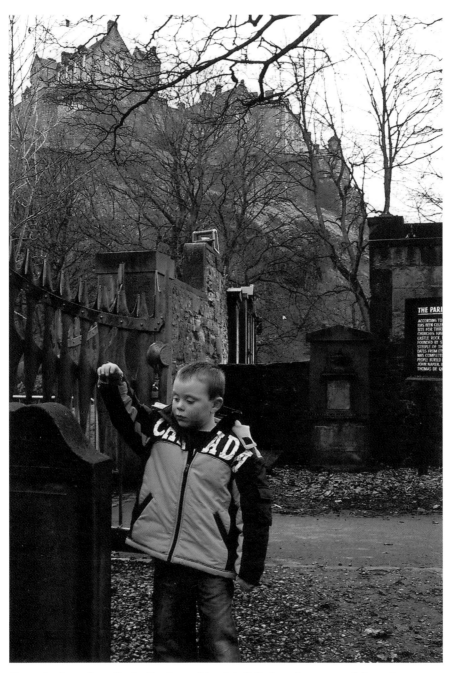

Deep in thought—Craig fascinated by this Edinburgh graveyard (2005).

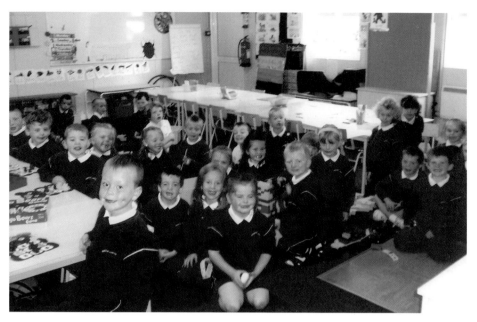

Craig with his classmates, Loreto Primary, Gorey.

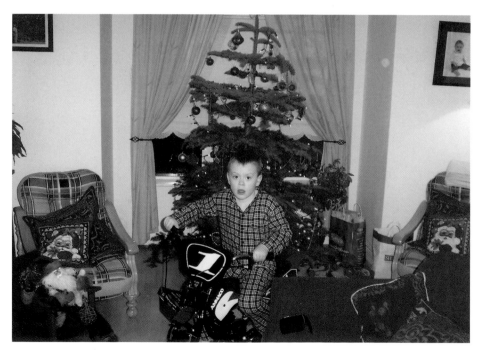

Craig's last ever Christmas with us (2005).

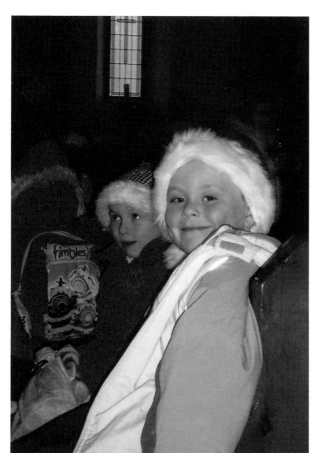

Craig at the Loreto School
Christmas Mass. He was
giddy with excitement that
day (Christmas 2005).

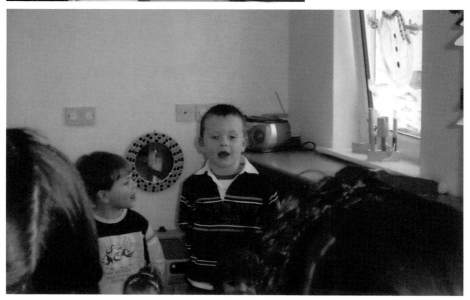

Craig carol-singing after his sterling nativity performance at Higgy's Montessori,
Gorey (Christmas 2005).

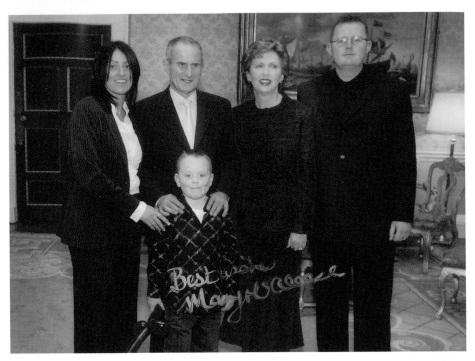

Posing with the President—attending the Christmas tree lighting ceremony at Áras an Uachtaráin (2005).

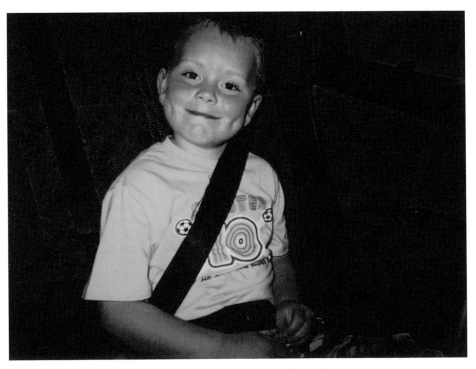

That wonderful smile—taken just a couple of months before the tumour was diagnosed (May 2006).

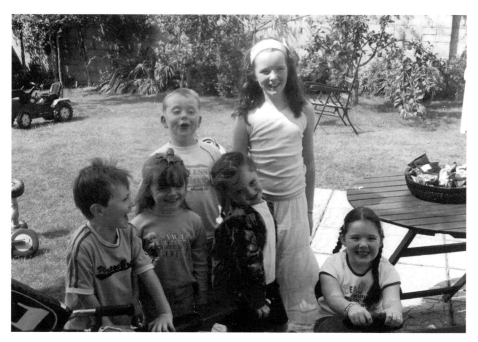

Craig with his cousins, Spot the Octopus … and Craig's mischievous ways (2006).

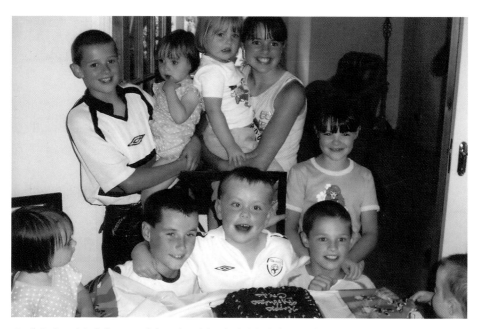

Craig's last birthday—celebrating his sixth birthday and posing with cousins (July 2006).

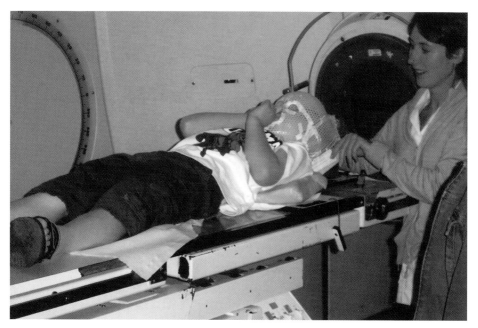

Our brave little man—the horrific daily ordeal of radiotherapy which Craig so bravely endured (summer 2006).

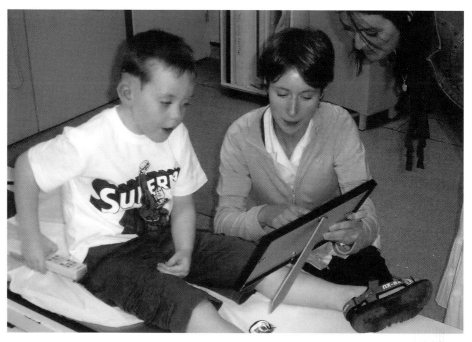

Craig receiving his bravery certificate and medal for completing his radiotherapy treatments (August 2006).

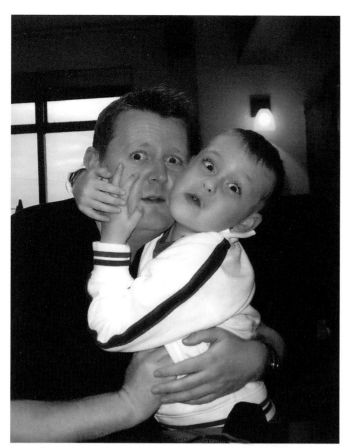

'Big hug for Daddy'—in a pub in Lahinch. Our first trip away after Craig's gruelling summer of radiotherapy (August 2006).

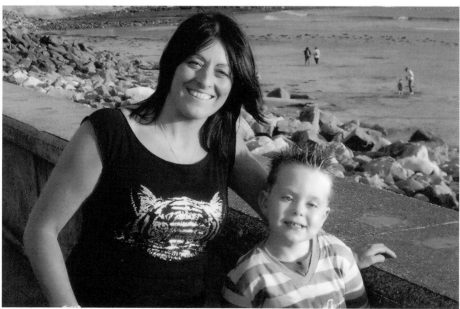

Craig and Mammy, Lahinch (August 2006).

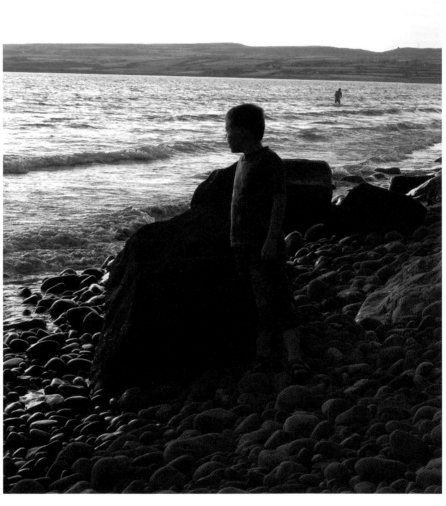

What lies ahead?—a poignant moment captured as Craig stares out to the Atlantic. He'd just finished his radiotherapy treatments (August 2006).

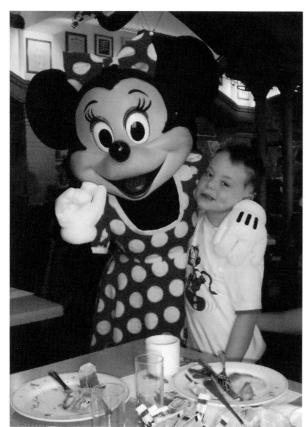

Craig having breakfast with Minnie Mouse at Disneyland Paris (2006).

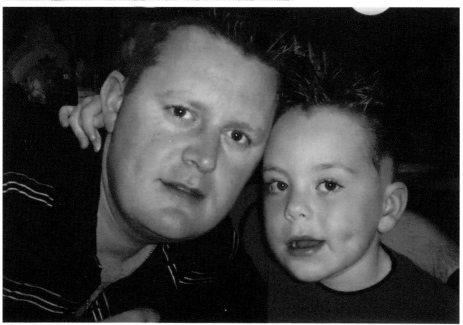

Daddy and Craig on holidays in Disneyland Paris, just weeks before he died (2006).

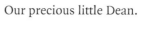
Our precious little Dean.

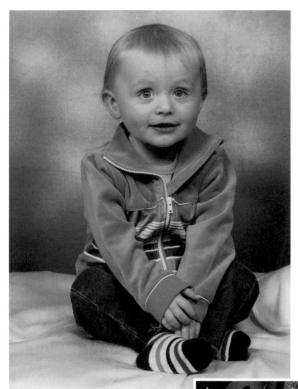

Dean saying hello to his big
brother at Craig's grave (2010).

the room and so while we all stood outside watching from a small TV screen, the sound of The Dubliners' 'You're drunk, you're drunk, you silly auld fool,' could be heard coming from within. When he was finished, the old man was clearly surprised to see such a young boy walking out. He looked at Craig, trying to reconcile his young years with the music he'd heard playing inside and then with a smile which hid his sadness said, 'There's a man who deserves a pint!' Craig smiled back at him and I could see the man shaking his head in disbelief. *Just a child.*

Craig's strength never failed to surprise us, though. He was incredible. I can still remember the morning he showed me, through his actions, just how strong he was.

We were about two weeks into Craig's radiotherapy treatment and as such had to travel up to St Luke's Hospital every day. At first, Craig found this impossible to do. The nausea and disorientation as he lay down flat was too much. 'It feels like I'm falling and the room is spinning,' he'd say, as he'd return to an upright position and gather his breath. 'I'm scared,' he'd continue, 'I can't do it.' The nervous tears would follow. But Craig was always so brave. He'd want a second or so to settle himself before asking either his mammy or me to hold his head as he leaned back. As he did so one of us would place our hands on either side of his head and hold him fast to the table. This is what he wanted. But it was a horrific ordeal each time. He would cry and hyperventilate as he looked us in the eye while we held him, and fought the urge to resurface. After about twenty or thirty seconds the dizzy spell would pass and he would be ok again, telling us 'It's stopped now'—but getting to that stage was such a trying ordeal for him. Never mind the plastic mask that had to be strapped tight to his face afterwards and which was then locked to the bed. The whole thing was a claustrophobe's nightmare and how he did it I'll never know. I know that I couldn't do what he did.

On this particular morning though Craig was at home in the bath getting washed and ready for the day ahead. We were due to go for his treatment later that morning and so we were all up early. I was outside getting a towel but when I returned I stopped still. Craig, who was previously sitting up in the bath, was now almost fully flat out, using his elbows for leverage. I moved over to sit on the toilet seat and watched him. His eyes darted to where I sat and he lunged forward, slight panic in his movement and with shortness in his breath.

'I nearly did it by myself,' he said, smiling. 'I was almost there, Daddy.'

'I could see that, Craig . . . Good man!' I was so moved. Barbara came into the room to see what he was doing and was almost tearful when she watched him. Craig kept trying and trying, each effort lasting a little longer than the last.

But the next day was the best. Again Craig was having his bath and I stayed with him as he once again tried to overcome the fear and nausea of lying back. But with each attempt he got a little braver. After a while I left the room to get some things in our bedroom. I was only in there about thirty seconds when I realised I couldn't hear any splashing noises. At that very same moment, I heard Craig calling me, 'Daddy!'

I raced back into the bathroom and the sight before me was perfect. Craig was lying out flat in the bath with the biggest smile on his face and his two beautiful blue eyes looking up at me. 'I did it!' he said, his dimples flashing up with the excitement that was his.

'Jesus, Craig, well done!' I said, as I reached in and patted him on the belly. 'Wait 'til I call your mammy,' I said. 'She wants to see this.'

'Well done, Craig!' Barbara beamed, as she came in and looked down on him. Kneeling, she then cupped the sides of his face and told him how strong he was.

It was such a picture to see Craig's smiling face emerging from a frame of white bubbles and to know in your heart what it took to do what he did. But Craig didn't leave it at that. He rose up again and after taking a few deep breaths forced himself to do it once more; and then again . . . and again . . . and again. It was remarkable. He was remarkable.

———

Coming up to the end of Craig's long run of gruelling treatment we decided that we all needed a break away. Poor Craig had never had a summer break at all. In his whole life in fact he'd never had a summer of freedom. Every year he'd been stuck in a crèche, while we both worked. This year was to be different, though. This year was to be his first; where he could get out and play with the other kids on the estate and enjoy a proper summer like all kids should. This year was supposed to be the first of many. Sadly, he never got that time.

But after everything Craig had been through, and what had been most certainly denied him, we wanted to give him something nice to look forward to; something to take his mind away from all the hospitals and doctors that had been plaguing his little life. We needed some straight-forward family time together and to fill it with as much fun and silliness as possible.

We decided on a trip to Lahinch in the end—we couldn't risk going abroad, given Craig's condition. But anywhere was better than where we'd been—anywhere there was to be no doctors, no hospitals, no mask and no radiation. So when we arrived in Lahinch we were greeted with the taste and smell of the fine ocean spray, the warmth of soft sandy beaches and the life-affirming energy of a strong Atlantic breeze. It was nature and it offered so much. In contrast to the clinical and the sterile, the wildness of it was so wonderful.

The days we spent there did so much for Craig and for us as a family. We escaped into a world where Craig was no longer a sick boy. We were allowed to be a family doing normal family things—a reprieve from the horrific and the unthinkable.

Returning from that trip we decided that Craig deserved so much more and so we decided it was time to bring him to Disneyland—he'd already told us this was where he wanted to go more than anywhere else.

Our time in Disneyland was among the very special times we got to spend as a family together. Just to see the happiness on Craig's face in spite of everything he was going through brought warmth and sunshine into our lives once again. He lived as a little boy, excited and happy, chasing from one magical thing to the next. He was a kid doing what all kids do and he loved every minute of it. As with our time in Lahinch we had all stepped out of our nightmare reality and into a place where everyone was safe and well and happy. Our other life could not touch us there. All was fine.

But reality is never one to be ignored and so as we boarded our flight home we knew we were inching ever closer to an uncertain future: a future that only promised one thing—the worst possible fear.

Chapter 6 ～

Weakening Hand, Loosening Grip

At the very beginning of October, Sunday 1 October in fact, Craig woke up and told us that he had a headache. He said that it felt 'weird'. When we asked him more about it he merely said, 'It feels like electricity on the right side of my face.' Neither Barbara nor I really knew what to make of it. If anything I wanted to believe it was something positive. Craig's face was already paralysed on that side and it was my hope that the 'electricity' he was feeling was perhaps the sensation coming back into it. The headache passed soon enough though and there was no real change in Craig's condition. Still, choosing to take this as a good sign I was a little more buoyant than expected.

The very next day Barbara and I decided to book a few days away for the three of us in Edinburgh. We'd been there the previous December and had such a great time. We knew it would give Craig, and indeed ourselves, something to look forward to and focus positively on.

So, without further ado I rang the Royal British Hotel and spoke with the man at reception. I made the booking for Thursday 2 November with a stay for three nights. Craig was delighted when he knew we were definitely going. He smiled that great smile of his and seemed energised with the anticipation.

As Craig walked around the house later that day both Barbara and I noticed something different about him. There was no denying it and all the joy of booking the trip was wiped out with the realisation. As he walked into the sitting room we could see how his right leg appeared to be dragging slightly. It wasn't severe or even immediately evident— but it was there. It was as though his right leg was that much heavier than the left that it had become slightly cumbersome. We asked Craig about it and he confirmed our fears. 'It just seems a bit funny,' was all that he said; was all that he wished to say, and no more. We didn't push it.

Another devastating blow; we were left feeling so incredibly scared. But we hid it, as always, and continued as normal. We remained positive and we focused on him getting through it. We prayed that the regular Essiac and Aloe Vera tinctures would be decisive in his recovering completely.

Craig continued to attend school, and with every day he did, we felt more encouraged and optimistic. He had endured a long summer of hospitals, sickness and loneliness; of being separated from other children and his friends. We knew Craig loved his school; his classmates. His closest friends—Andrew, Ciaran, Dylan, Michael and Mathew—were so important to him. We'd hear these names being mentioned so often.

One day while Craig was at school we even decided to drive up by the school gates just to peek in and see how he was getting on during his lunch break. Moving slowly past, there he was, standing in the midst of four other boys, gesturing with his arms as they all watched and listened intently. We were just so relieved to see that he wasn't struggling or being left out. In fact, he was right in the thick of it, being as strong as ever.

About a day or so after that we called up, as normal, to collect Craig from school. We arrived, walking through the gates and down to the yard area where all the prefabs were arranged. Normally all of us parents would stand out in the central yard, just outside our relevant prefabs, and wait for our children to spill out. However, as we entered the main yard area that afternoon we could see that Craig's entire class were already outside. It was obvious that they were still finishing up their PE lesson. Barbara and I, along with the other parents, stood nearby and watched on as the kids were assembled in several queues, each with a large circular ring a number of metres ahead of them. One by one the kids were taking their turn in trying to toss a bean bag into the circular ring ahead of them. We could see Craig in the queue and we knew his turn was coming soon. We felt for him. We knew that his vision and coordination were so severely compromised that this otherwise ordinary challenge was now a monstrous one for him.

When his turn came we prayed that he would get it in. We could feel the expectation, the empathy, of the other parents around us as Craig lined up the bean bag in his hand and stared awkwardly at the target ahead. He had to look diagonally to compensate for the other eye. *C'mon, Craig you can do it!* we thought, gritting our teeth as we watched on. Craig pulled his arm back and swung it gently back and forth, gauging his power, and then with a final flourish and with his tongue sticking out he lobbed it into the air . . . it went straight in. *Thank God!* I thought as a lump filled my throat.

Barbara and I clapped on excitedly as we watched his fellow classmates shout 'Yeeaaahh, good one, Craig!' and as he smiled, raising his arm in the air in victory. He glanced over in our direction and looked so smitten. We were incredibly proud of him. We both just wanted to run over, hug him and lift him into the air . . . which we did, just after the class was dismissed.

That memory continues to be a very poignant one for us; one that brings tears of pride and smiles of joy for how Craig triumphed over the obstacles that lay in his path. It was a bright, sunny autumnal day too and so the image of Craig's raised arm and smiling face as the sun shone through his golden hair and while his friends cheered him on is quite possibly one of the most uplifting visual memories we have of that dark time. If only we'd had a camera at that moment it would have captured a most precious and spectacularly important image. But we have it in our heads; that's more important. We can look at it any time we want, day or night, and we can see and hear the joy that he felt over and over again, and be happy for him for that moment.

———

Craig and I loved the woods. There's no doubt about it. We both found something magical in the shelter of its dark and verdant surrounds. It was a place of mystique, brimming with all things natural and serene. We'd often go for our long walks together, checking out the wildlife and flora that lined our path. We'd walk along talking, thinking and messing as we found fun and laughter in each other's company and in the spoils of nature's bounty. But not all our trips were so light and free. Some are a little more difficult to reminisce upon . . .

He Ain't Heavy . . . He's My Son

Craig was always full of energy as we rambled through the forests. He'd run ahead to check out some stick or funny looking tree or gape into some pond-like puddle. Sometimes he'd hide and then call out to me (more often than not I'd see exactly where he'd gone, but I'd of course play the fool anyway). I'd call out in reply but deliberately look away from where he was. Doing this I could nearly always see him in my periphery, occasionally peeking out from behind some tree or shrubbery, and then watch as he'd move to another spot. I'd usually play along with this and let him 'win' so to speak but every now and then—just to spice things up—I'd take a different approach. Whilst catching him in my periphery, and knowing that he was staring right at me, I'd freakishly and totally unexpectedly sprint immediately towards him shouting 'I'm gonna get ye!! I'm gonna get ye!!' I'd laugh to myself, watching him shaking—a curious combination of terror, shock and giddiness having seized him. He'd stand frozen for a couple of seconds before screeching 'Oh Jesus! . . .' then turn on his heels and leg it. I'd continue shouting while getting closer and closer and listen as Craig's nervous laughter anticipated my snatching him at any second. When I'd eventually catch up, I'd let out a final high-pitched roar, then grab him under his arms and swing him around in a circle.

Craig was always electrified by this; he'd fizz with uncontrollable energy and become intensely animated. I suppose, from his perspective, it was akin to the feeling one might have on safari where at one moment you, the ignorant tourist, are staring at an elephant who is quietly going about his business—eating some foliage perhaps—but who then turns and charges you down. You find yourself unexpectedly scrambling for your life upon increasingly weakening and rubbery limbs, and with the downy micro-hairs on your neck tingling with sheer panic, you simply cannot escape the terrifying sound of immense biomass crunching and snapping vegetation as it bears down on you. Every biological function in your body compels you to run away and yet your brain tells you that you will be caught—the rapidly approaching carnage of toothed bulk and momentum behind proving too much for the great abacus within to ignore. Part of you wants, yearns, to just give up and surrender to the jelly limbs that have already failed you. How easy it would be to just shut down and collapse in a heap of pathetic surrender . . . Now, I can't be certain, but Craig may have felt something like that as I chased him.

All I know is that we had such great fun and adventure whenever we were in the woods. Running, walking, chasing, hiding, exploring, finding and even learning: it was all part of the experience. Under every log there were wonders to be seen; standing on the bridge looking to the river below we'd witness glorious living treasures swerving and skating above and below its earthy flow. Beneath fallen leaves and across the living, all manner of things could be discovered, each holding our gaze and fascination as we talked about the thing before us. But mostly it was just being with each other; spending that time as father and son in a place that we both enjoyed. And that's what made it so very hard when things began to change.

Initially I had begun to notice how Craig was not his usual self as we moved through the woods. This was ok though—he was sick and had endured so much with his treatments and medication that it was entirely understandable. We'd wander around with the same exuberant conversation and enthusiasm but just not with the same physical energy. The walks were more leisurely and less intense: no more chasing or hiding, just talking and walking. I wasn't worried though. I could reason and account for it. I figured that when he improved everything would be back to normal. *All in good time; just be patient.*

Besides, I was really enjoying the conversations we were having; there was something deeper, more earnest about them. I recall how on one occasion Craig asked me to bring his penknife to the woods. (This was a penknife that Craig found in the surrounding grounds of St Luke's Hospital. He and his Uncle Darren, who had come to see him get his treatment that day, had run off to hide among the many trees and discovered it there.) So, on this day in the woods Craig and I strolled along as normal before coming to a section near the river where a tree trunk lay on its side, providing a welcome seat. Craig was asking me how people survived a long time ago when they had to live outside in the woods with no electricity or houses, so as I explained I decided I'd show him how (sort of). I told him that they used to fish in the rivers and hunt wild animals for their meat and fur. I took a stick from the ground and began carving a sharpened end onto it with the penknife and then stood to demonstrate how the 'cavemen' would have crept up on the wild animals and hurled the spear at them.

'Did cavemen have penknives?' Craig asked me, his sarcasm obvious. I laughed.

'No, smart arse,' I replied, looking at him smiling up at me. 'They would have used flint—a type of sharp stone—to either carve or put on the end of the stick as a spearhead.' Craig seemed happy enough with this—the sarcastic look melting away.

I also picked up another stick and bent it into a bow shape. I showed him how they would have made bows and arrows and we talked about hunting, making fire and building homes from the branches and leaves. Craig was really interested and it struck me how pleasant it was to be sitting there just blabbering on about all this stuff. He really wanted to know. He was mesmerised as we both journeyed together into a world of wild men, spears and hunting.

While we sat there I looked over at a tree that stood at the corner of an ascending path up through the woods.

'Let's carve our names into that tree,' I said to Craig, pointing it out in front of me.

'Yeah!' Craig was thrilled at the idea.

We walked over and as we picked out our spot we kept looking around us to make sure nobody else was approaching from the other directions. We picked a side of the bark that didn't face out onto the path—making it instantly a more secretive, hidden marking that only we knew of. When Craig told me the coast was clear I began carving. It simply read:

CRAIG

+

DADDY

2006

As I carved it I fantasised how wonderful, how truly magical it would be, for Craig and me to come back to this spot in years to come and see it there—a forever reminder of this day. The implied positivity was something that lifted my heart and gave me hope. I felt it was a bold, determined action—a physicalised affirmation of my belief in Craig and in his survival.

————

It was moments like this that were so special to me, and although we had enjoyed many such times over the years, there was something extra special about those more leisurely ambles. There was something deeper and more profound in Craig's presence as we shared those gentle jaunts along wooded paths. As the weeks rolled by, however, Craig was clearly becoming weaker.

Our last time together in the woods was heartbreaking for me. We'd been at home and I'd asked Craig if he was interested in going for a walk.

'Yeah,' he said, looking happy to be getting out of the house.

'We'll just do a short walk,' I said, knowing that he probably wasn't up to anything more.

'Okay,' he said, as he put his white cardigan on over his t-shirt and got ready.

We drove out to the woods and parked in our usual spot, before climbing out and walking to the main entrance. I walked slowly, noticing that Craig was walking unusually slowly. About ten metres into our walk I looked at Craig and could see something wasn't right. He looked back at me and with heavy eyes said, 'Daddy, will you carry me?'

'Of course I will. Come here,' I said, leaning down to pick him up and lifting him up to my head height. Craig's legs hung limp around my waist and as we moved forward on the path he put his arms around me with his head slowly sinking into the nape of my neck. I could hear him shallow breathing—he was exhausted. I walked a little further along, but Craig wasn't speaking. The fear in me began to rupture. I wondered what was going through his mind. Was he depressed? His body letting him down again like that. Was he doing this for me? He knew how much I loved going to the woods with him; was he pushing on just for my sake? I spoke:

'Do you want to head home, Craig?' I asked. 'We can wait until your energy returns again, okay?'

'Okay,' was all he could muster.

He had walked only a few metres and was drained. The implication terrified me and all I wanted to do was cry. I hated that this illness was advancing on him, taking away all the things that he enjoyed. I carried him in my arms back to the car and we drove back home. As we came through the door Barbara looked at us both and then directly at me. She knew something was wrong and her heart fell. Craig made his way into the sitting room and sat up on the couch to watch TV while Barbara and I went in to the kitchen. I told her how weak Craig had been. Neither of us wanted to believe that Craig was slipping, but we felt it. It destroyed us to watch him being robbed of the few things he had left. I wanted to scream at the world for being so fucking cruel to an innocent little boy.

Mid-way through October Craig's school Principal, Sister Breda, came over to speak with us. Having spoken with Adrienne, the teacher's assistant who sat with Craig every day, she wanted to voice her concern over Craig's apparent diminishing balance. Adrienne had noticed that Craig was faltering on his feet slightly and was a little concerned that this may eventually pose a problem for him. He also had developed a bad cough. Sister Breda had echoed this concern and felt she needed to bring it to our attention. She was quick to highlight that they were perfectly open to keeping Craig in school—in fact they welcomed it— but they'd have to monitor his situation and perhaps have to consider other options were Craig's condition to diminish further.

She was perfectly correct of course. It wouldn't serve Craig well at all to be so poorly in school, and of course the school itself had its own responsibilities to consider too. Sister Breda was always so considerate and thoughtful when handling the situation and we could always see the honesty and emotion in her eyes when she spoke. She thought a lot of Craig. He had worked his magic on her too, it seems. But for us, hearing any kind of 'defeatist' talk at that time pained us deeply. Of course it wasn't defeatist in the least, merely practical and born out of true heart-felt concern, but nonetheless it hurt. The truth frequently does, I suppose. We wanted to hear that Craig was still flying; that he continued to excel despite all the odds. But that simply wasn't so . . .

The following morning we brought Craig to see the doctor who confirmed that Craig had an ear and throat infection. Our first reaction was one of relief and of renewed hope. Maybe this ear infection was causing Craig's balance problems, and would pass; nothing to do with his tumour at all. After speaking with our liaison and palliative nurses we began Craig on a higher dose (4 mg) of his dexamethasone anti-inflammatory medication. I hoped that this was just a temporary measure until the infection cleared and that all would be back to normal within a few days.

The next day we decided to keep Craig home from school to give him a chance to recuperate properly. We took him to Glendalough to get some good fresh air and, with Craig sitting reluctantly in the wheelchair that we'd brought with us, we roamed around for a short while. Every now and then Craig would get back out of the chair, but not for long. He wasn't able. His legs weren't up to it. It was so frightening to see.

A few days later, on the Friday in fact, we returned to the doctor to see if the infection had lifted. Unfortunately he confirmed that it was still there and so prescribed some stronger erythromycin antibiotics. We left hoping that they would do the trick, and soon. Craig's balance and walking were suffering and we desperately wanted to see him back to normal. We wanted to see if it *was* the infection that was giving rise to Craig's latest symptoms, and not something altogether more sinister. We didn't even want to contemplate that.

The following week began well, with Craig staying in school for the entire Monday. He was, despite the ongoing infection, in rather good form. The following morning we returned to our GP, Dr Breslin, who confirmed that the infection was still there and prescribed a third antibiotic to try and counter it. Apart from the hampered walking, Craig was still in good form so, after discussing it with the doctor and with Craig, we took him to school. Craig wanted to be with his friends and was eager to get back. However, later that morning the school rang us and told us that Craig's temperature was quite high and they thought it best that he go home.

When we collected Craig he was upset. He didn't want to go home. He wanted to stay with his pals. As before, despite the raised temperature, Craig was feeling strong and didn't see why he had to go home. He thought it was so unfair that he was the only one being made to leave and to be honest Barbara and I were a little annoyed too. We knew that the time he spent with his friends was very important to him, and *for* him, and it was so much more beneficial that he stayed. But the school took that decision and we went along with it. Theirs was a practical and precautionary decision, and they were of course perfectly right to take it. It was just a shame.

The very next morning Craig's temperature returned to normal and so he spent the entire day in school. We took this opportunity to sneak up the town and to go all out in buying a stack of Halloween decorations. We spent the first half of the morning shopping around for all the stuff and then the other half hanging it all up in the house. We bought ghoulish headstones, ghostly figures, giant rats and monsters that we hung on the walls. We even bought a large, almost life-size witch that we placed in a standing position in a box at the top of the stairs. Beneath her we strategically placed a camping lamp that cast menacing shadows about her grotesque features and which gave her a terrifying appearance when viewed from the front door. We had all manner of wonderfully spooky puppets and dolls dangling and dotted around the rooms and it looked positively magical.

When we collected Craig from school and he walked through the doors the first words that came out of his mouth were 'Wow . . . Cool!' He was so excited. We walked around the house as he examined all the different bits and pieces with his face lighting up the more he saw. But the witch really stole the show. She looked intensely scary as her face took on a gaunt, deathly look from the eerie shadows cast from the lamp below . . . Craig loved her. He loved the whole setup: 'Thank you, Mammy. Thank you, Daddy,' he said, as he hugged us both. We couldn't have hoped for a better reaction.

The following morning we returned to the doctor who finally gave Craig the all-clear on the infection. His ear and throat were back to normal and the rattle in his chest was gone. Craig returned to school after his visit and spent the whole day there. But Barbara and I were growing ever more concerned. Craig's balance and walking certainly hadn't returned to normal and so it clearly wasn't the infection that was causing it.

That night Craig awoke with a terrible headache and in the morning he was violently ill. There was no way he was going to school that day, so we kept him home and looked after him. His headache and sickness passed but his balance was almost completely shot. He simply could not walk unaided and we were devastated. He had to call us each time he needed to move and we'd have to hold his hand as he tried desperately to co-ordinate his legs.

The next day his condition deteriorated even further. He could not walk at all and his left arm wouldn't move properly. He was very sick and the speed of his deterioration was frightening. Barbara and I were left absolutely terrified. As always, in the mornings he'd warn us that he was going to get sick and wait for us to fetch the basin before doing so. But increasingly these vomiting episodes were being accompanied by blistering headaches. Craig would cry out, the sheer pain and nausea overwhelming him, and yet there was little that we could do except to hold him; to let him know we were with him through it. The medication would then be adjusted to try and combat these episodes but still they seemed to happen.

One morning after a particularly horrendous episode Craig just cried out, 'Why me? Why is this happening to me?' as he struggled with the overbearing pain and suffering that had become his life. He cried out over and over again, with the basin under his chin and his arm holding his head. He sounded utterly defeated. All we could do was hold him and kiss him and reassure him that everything would be ok soon, as we fought to hide the tears that rolled down our cheeks. I simply cannot describe the torment we felt watching our child crying out, pleading for mercy as he was slowly tortured before our eyes.

But Craig was so unfathomably strong—stronger than us for sure. His dips were brief and through it all he remained impossibly good spirited. He seemed to take it largely in his stride. When the bouts of sickness and pain would finally pass, his humour—that sharp wit of his—would emerge once again. Every time he was knocked down he would get back up. He took his limitations and rolled with them.

Craig's condition was such at this point that returning to school would require him being in a wheelchair. We knew Craig wasn't fond of the wheelchair and so sat him down to speak about it. Craig, as always, knew his own mind. He made it absolutely and immediately clear to us that he did not want to go back to school in 'that thing'. We understood. We put his mind at ease straight away and told him that was fine. *We would have to teach Craig from home ourselves.*

——

On 21 October—my father's birthday—Craig was tested once more but once again his inner strength shone through. We had pre-organised to go out for a meal in Gorey to mark the occasion, but when the day came Craig was extremely ill. His recent deterioration had been rapid. He had been throwing up quite a bit and was very weak indeed. The effects of the tumour were pulling his little life apart and the constant sickness and bodily decline left him feeling frail and frightened.

On the day in question we had suggested to Craig over and over again that it might be a better idea to just get a takeaway and relax in the comfort of the house instead of going out. We didn't want him to feel under pressure about going out when he was so sick. We tried our best to make it sound like we were doing it for our own reasons and not because of Craig, but he wouldn't hear of it. He was determined to go out and celebrate his granddan's birthday properly, despite how he was feeling.

We had already picked a birthday card together so later on that evening Craig told me to fetch it for him. He said he wanted to write on the card himself and so we pulled up at the dining room table and sat to write out his message. As Craig began to write I could see his arms and hand shaking. The nerves in the muscles were not firing right and so he struggled to control his writing hand. I sat there and watched as his handwriting scrawled uncontrollably across the card. My heart bled as he began to cry with frustration. He just couldn't keep his hand from shaking. I tried to help him but he said he wanted to do it by himself. He cried out of anger and disappointment as the results of his writing looked so ragged and unlike his normal hand. I asked him whether he wanted me to finish it for him, but he cried out in anger saying he wanted to do it all by himself. It killed me to see him have to go through this but his strength of character dazzled me. It was clear that this was one of the most difficult things for him to do but he never once entertained the thought of giving up. Despite the anguish and the hurt he was feeling he wanted to see it through. When he finished it he just put his head down and began crying so hard. 'Granddan is going to hate this . . . my writing is so ugly,' he sobbed, feeling so embarrassed by the alien scrawl that lay in front of him.

'I can tell you one thing, Craig,' I said, jumping in straight away to soothe his pain, 'Granddan is going to absolutely cherish that card more than any other card you've ever given him.'

'No, he's not,' he whimpered. 'He's going to think it's so baby writing.'

'He certainly won't, Craig,' I said. 'Granddad knows that the lump in your head is making your hand shake and when he sees this card he's going to be so proud of how you could still write it for him. He's going to know how strong you are for being able to get your words written and he's going to feel so happy that you did it for him.'

'No, he won't,' Craig mumbled under his breath.

'Oh yes, he will.'

'Will he?'

'I guarantee it, Craig. I'm going to tell him how I watched you fight your way through and how proud I was to see you beat that lump.'

Craig softened after this, but I could see in his eyes that the shaking had worried him. I knew that he was so annoyed that he couldn't do what he wanted to do.

My mother and father arrived down later that evening and Craig looked concerned at the moment his granddan went to open the card. I waited until my father opened the card and read it before telling him just how strong Craig had been to fight through the shakes. I could see, just by looking at my father's face as he read the card, that he was very deeply touched.

He walked straight over to Craig and gave him a great big hug and a kiss saying, 'Thank you for such a beautiful card and for writing those lovely words, Craig.' Craig smiled and you could see a certain amount of relief in his face. 'I know how hard that must have been, Craig,' he continued, 'and I feel very privileged that you did that for me!' Craig looked even better after hearing that.

Some months later my father told us that he was so moved by that card that he was taking it to the grave with him. He said it was the most special card he had ever received in his life, as it made him feel so very special for receiving it.

When we were all ready we headed up to the restaurant, parking just outside. I had to carry Craig in and we were lucky to get a nice table at the window. Barbara went through the menu with Craig and helped him to choose something he liked. He wanted spaghetti Bolognese in fact. A few minutes later plates of food began arriving at the table. It all smelled delicious. When Craig got his he took a spoonful and sat back. But then he started to hyperventilate and whimper. He cried as he panicked, saying 'Oh no, I'm going to be sick, Mammy, I'm sorry.' Barbara grabbed his shoulders and just told him to get sick where he was and not worry about it. Craig had always been so careful about being sick into a basin that he hated the idea of getting sick on the floor. But he did. He leaned downwards and got sick under the table. His poor little stomach was just so sensitive and the first taste of the meal had made him feel nauseous. We tried to calm him down as wave after wave of sickness struck him.

When he was done he looked so embarrassed and upset, believing that he had ruined the birthday meal. We told him that it wasn't his fault at all and not to worry about it for a second. He looked very drawn and weak and we asked him whether he wanted to go home instead. He just quietly nodded his head and said 'Yes'. He had tried his very hardest to come out with us, to make the day special, but he was just too ill.

Back at the house we laid Craig out on the couch, and he looked relieved to be home. But despite the sickness he had felt he said he was starving. The course of anti-inflammatory tablets he was on always gave him a ferocious if unpredictable appetite. It seemed like every day fluctuated with extremes of intense hunger and heavy sickness. I quickly rustled up some chicken noodles and made them into sandwiches for him . . . and he devoured the lot. We all stood in the sitting room and smiled as he munched and savoured every mouthful.

But deeper inside there was a knowing that what just happened was not good. It whispered fear into our very souls and everyone who stood in that room felt it too, I'm sure. Everyone seemed to be looking at Craig and smiling, but their eyes told a different tale. There was a pity and a sense of hopelessness in that room that chilled deep into my bones and I couldn't breathe with it. It felt like Craig was slipping away before our very eyes and there was nothing that anyone could do but watch.

But for every new inch that the illness gained, we saw in Craig a towering spirit of resolve and strength. Yes, that night Craig got sick in the restaurant. Yes, he suffered the apparent indignity of it and of not being able to neatly write a card to his granddan. But that's not what I choose to remember about that night. What I remember is how Craig sat at that table and persevered through the pain and the shame. I can still see the tears and hear him cry, but all the while with his head down and his hand still moving across the card. I remember that Craig *made* it to the restaurant. Despite the illness and the weakness and how easy it would have been for him to say *No, I'm not up to it*, he pushed himself for others. So for what the illness took physically, it served only to reveal the raw majesty of Craig's soul and the true dignity with which he carried himself. That is what I remember.

————

What do you do when your child is scared? What can you possibly say when those little eyes meet yours and in them you see the fear that you hoped would never be there; when they pierce your soul, crying out for *you* to help them—and there is nothing you can do.

Craig's spirit is a strong one. It always has been and always will be. People often equate strength with fearlessness. This is wholly wrong. True strength can only ever be shown in the face of fear; in feeling it and overcoming it. This is why Craig's spirit is so strong.

On more than one occasion, but only very rarely, Craig would wobble. How could he not? He was no fool. He had an intuitive way that we often overlooked; wanted to overlook perhaps. Barbara and I both had individual experiences with Craig where he seemed to speak from a place of knowing: a place where his fears seemed to bubble to the surface and, helpless to stop them, he'd be overcome . . .

'I'm Dying, Amn't I?'

I remember one evening while putting Craig to bed and going through our ritual of prayers how he so quietly said something that left me horrified. We had actually finished all our prayers and our messing around and were talking about his soldiers—I used to tell Craig to imagine, as often as he could, that he had thousands of soldiers inside in his body that were slowly but surely killing off the lump in his head, making it smaller and smaller. This night, as we began to discuss them, Craig sighed forcefully. He looked fed up— bored of talking about the bloody soldiers and I couldn't blame him. But it was more than just being bored or fed up. He looked away from me, to the wall behind, and said 'I'm dying, amn't I?'

I was stunned but couldn't allow a pause. 'Of course you're not, darlin',' I replied instantly. 'What makes you say that?' Several thoughts raced through my mind. What did make him say that? Did a child in school mention something about tumours and dying, maybe after overhearing their parents? What do I say to him? How do I make his fear go away?

'I am. I know I am,' he continued, and then a stream of tears came.

I reached in and hugged him close, then stared straight into his eyes. 'Look at me, Craig. You're not dying, do you hear me!' It was the truth as far as I was concerned. I didn't believe he was going to die. Craig was so remarkable I believed that he'd pull through it. I believed that he was the rare exception—that he would be the miracle case. The Aloe Vera we were giving him; the Essiac solution; Craig's strength.

'I am, I'm always sick, it's not getting better,' he cried up at me, my heart drowning with every word he uttered. His tear-soaked eyes looked up at me, stealing the wind from my lungs and tightening my throat.

I tried desperately to calm him. I looked at him and smiled (it killed me) and told him with a giggle, 'You're not dying. Jaysus, I'll be dead long before you.' Craig looked at me and the beginnings of a little smile crept across his lips.

'No you won't!' he said with a sniffle, as he rubbed his eyes.

'Of course I will!' I asserted strongly, almost comically, as I sought to dilute his fears even further. 'That fucking lump is just making you sick but its days are numbered, I tell ye!'

Craig chuckled as I swore. He loved to hear the F word, and I loved to make him laugh. Now was especially important and I knew when he laughed that he was calm again. I was relieved.

We spoke for a little while after that, as he calmed further, and I made sure I swore and made him laugh as much as I could. I couldn't bear to think that he was contemplating his own death. My stomach was sick knowing that his mind was perhaps understanding his situation, maybe giving up when there was so much—everything—to fight for. I wanted him to let go of those thoughts and embrace hope and belief in being well again.

When I left the room that night, Craig was smiling at me. The darker thoughts were gone and he was, I hoped, in some way assured again. I walked into my back room, put my hands over my face—like a child—and cried. After a moment or so I exhaled, wiped my eyes and walked back downstairs to Barbara. I told her what Craig had said and she cried too. The pain was incredible.

But the next morning Craig woke up to fight on and, without a thought for the night before, he smiled and laughed his way through yet another day of sickness, confinement and loneliness . . . A remarkable little man, the strongest I've ever known.

The day after my father's birthday we decided to take Craig out of the house to get some fresh air. We took him down for a walk along the road front in Courtown and as it was incredibly cold we were all dressed in our warmest wears. Craig was by now totally wheelchair bound. Within only a few days he had fallen so fast. We walked along the road that led from the harbour to the woods, wheeling Craig in front of us as we moved against the bitter wind that bit into us. Craig was completely covered up with a jacket, hat and scarf and was unnervingly quiet as we strolled along. We tried nattering away as we moved but Craig's answers or contributions were always monosyllabic. *We knew he was feeling low.*

Steadily his silence grew and that walk became one of the coldest, most disheartening and painful walks that I've ever had to endure. The quiet of it. The sorrow of it. And then it got worse. I looked down and could hear Craig whimpering . . . and then I saw why. He was struggling with his left hand, trying desperately to put it into his jacket pocket and out of the freezing cold. Barbara and I, who'd seen this, reacted instantly, placing it in for him. It was ice cold to the touch. *How long had it been out; how long had he struggled before we noticed?* I never felt as low as I did in that moment. We all felt so beaten. But with that feeling came the need to fight back. Barbara and I tried our best to raise Craig's spirits and stoke that powerful fire of his, but although he perked up a little it was clear to see he was still holding back.

Eventually we ran out of road and so had to turn around and double back. Craig remained unusually, but understandably, introspective as we made our way back along the same road. We knew that he was embarrassed being in that wheelchair. We knew that he was most likely nervous about bumping into one of his friends from school and feeling ashamed of his situation. But even in that Craig's bravery was shining through. He knew that he would be in that wheelchair when we asked him to go for a walk back at the house. He could have moped—and Christ who could blame him—and refused to go. He could have felt sorry for himself and risked nothing by staying where he was. But no. He faced his limits, his situation and the world by getting out there. Not many could do the same. Jesus, I've stayed in when I've had a bloody cold sore, never mind being sickened, crippled and deformed by a ruthless tumour. Craig earned everyone's respect for the sheer strength of his character, and so as difficult as it was to walk along with Craig while he was so very ill and so incredibly low, we were the two proudest parents in the world and our love for him couldn't have been stronger.

Just as we were almost back to where we started we happened to look to our right and were surprised to see my parents and my sister Mel walking over a bridge towards us. They hadn't rung us, or arranged to meet—indeed they didn't even know we'd be there. They had called down and when we weren't at the house just chanced to see if we were in Courtown. They literally walked into us.

Craig looked over and we could sense his embarrassment. As they came towards us Craig remained withdrawn. They had never seen him in the wheelchair before and he felt uncomfortable.

They came over saying hello to Craig as normal and making no fuss about the wheelchair at all. This seemed to put Craig somewhat at ease, but still he was quiet. We walked along together in the direction of the harbour but it was only while we stopped and Mel bent down to talk to him that Craig's spirit emerged forcefully once more. He leaned into Mel's face and, what had appeared at first to be a long exaggerated kiss, was soon revealed to be a ploy for him to rub his snotty running nose into her face. Mel pulled back, laughing at the cheek of him. It was a beautiful moment—seeing Craig's wit and devilment back in business as he climbed out from beneath the shadow and dazzled us yet again with his light. The joy we felt witnessing that cheeky little smile on his face was something else. If ever a single act could so completely transform an atmosphere it was then. Craig had turned it around and flipped it on its head.

Just about then Barbara's mother and sister Shirley arrived in Courtown to meet us too, so we all went for a coffee nearby. Craig was starving (as always) so I nipped across to the chippers and fetched him a burger. We sat there together chatting away as Craig devoured the deliciously hot rounded loveliness that steamed enticingly, but briefly, before him. He remained buoyant as we sat there enjoying that special time together and so what began as a grim and uneasy afternoon had, unexpectedly, ended up as a thoroughly pleasant evening.

—

With Craig now so severely incapacitated by the progression of his illness all hopes for a camping trip that we had planned earlier had to be abandoned. Craig's condition was rapidly deteriorating, with his left arm now curled up towards his face as the muscles permanently contracted. His speech had gone so bad that he sounded exhausted as he tried to communicate. His words were slow and laboured, and very nasal sounding. He was increasingly sick and suffered terrible headaches. It was soul destroying to watch him endure so much.

During that week the Crumlin liaison nurse, Fiona, called down to see us. She was accompanied by Anne Gortland, Craig's palliative nurse. What Fiona told us that day left us numb. She talked us through prescriptions for morphine and various muscle relaxants for probable seizures that Craig would have as his illness progressed. She told us how to administer the drugs and what to do when a seizure occurs. I was speechless. The picture she painted was one so horrendous that I feared were I to open my mouth I would burst into tears. Barbara was stronger. She reacted for both of us. I merely nodded, saying little or nothing at all as far as I can remember. While we were speaking with Fiona, Anne had gone into the sitting room to distract and occupy Craig. Unfortunately, and unusually, Craig had become very upset while Anne was with him. Craig knew Anne quite well from all her visits so this was a surprise to hear him crying so hard. The combination of what we'd just been told and hearing Craig's cry was overwhelming. We just wanted to race in and grab Craig and run away from all this pain. Our rational minds understood everything we were being told but our emotional sides just wanted to get away from all these people with their talk of sickness and failure. We felt so protective of Craig and couldn't wait for them to just leave and let us be. Their mere presence heralded doom and I certainly couldn't stand it anymore. I can't remember how we conducted ourselves that day exactly—I expect it wasn't with warmth or with any measure of welcoming. But we simply had nothing to give. Our world was ending with every word they spoke and all tolerance was gone.

When they left I was a beaten man. Of the two of us, I had always been the optimistic one. I always believed that Craig was going to get through it. Barbara wanted to believe, but deep down inside she knew. I wrestled with my fears every day but I held onto my belief with both hands and never let go. I couldn't stomach the alternative. But when those nurses left they had worked my fingers free. They had spoken with an ominous, familiar knowing that had unhinged me. I was terrified.

Barbara, Craig and I just hugged each other after they'd gone. We sat together in that sitting room and prayed for time to stand still. Neither Barbara nor I could take our eyes off Craig. We watched as he ate his food; as he watched the TV; as he did everything. I couldn't speak for the rest of that day. Barbara rang her mother to tell her the news; something I couldn't do. I knew I'd break down on the phone; that the words wouldn't come. Barbara rang and told them instead.

The next day we took Craig to Lynhams Hotel, in Laragh, Co. Wicklow . . .

Chapter 7 ~
Letting Go

There are very few times that stand out in my mind as strongly as the day we brought Craig up to Lynhams Hotel. It is a memory that is at once filled with such bitter sadness and with such triumphant happiness that it seems to capture the essence of Craig and his journey through life.

My brother Darren had just come over from England to see Craig and we had all arranged to meet up for some food in Lynhams Hotel. Craig was looking forward to seeing his uncle but Barbara and I knew there was something different about Craig's demeanour. He seemed to be very subdued, very quiet in himself. His illness was visibly taking its toll but we knew it was more than this. Craig's spirit had always been strong and positive and with Darren coming home he was usually bursting with excitement. But this time he looked troubled. He never said anything to us and before we left we made sure he genuinely wanted to go. But he was worried. The last time he had seen Darren, he was in better shape. He was walking and running everywhere—not in some stupid wheelchair. He'd run down the hospital corridor to meet and hug his uncle, almost running through him. His face had been normal and he could talk properly. He had been so full of energy that despite his sickness he pushed himself to jump up and down on his birthday bouncy castle all day. Maybe Craig remembered all this . . . and was nervous. Maybe he just didn't know what Darren would think of him: sitting in a wheelchair unable to walk, a badly contorted and swollen face paralysed on one side, and an inability to speak in the voice that had always been his. I just think Craig felt embarrassed.

The drive up to Laragh had been uneasy. Craig was sitting in the back, snuggled in beside his mammy, and he was quiet. I could see him in the rear-view mirror as he looked out the window and it pained me to think what was going through his mind. We tried talking excitedly about seeing Darren and about what we'd have to eat when we got there, but always there was this holding back. I'm sure he just wished that he was well again, just his old self, and not this crippled version. I'm sure he was angry and sad and self-conscious.

When we got to Laragh we turned into the car park at Lynhams and as we drove down to find a place we passed my parents and Darren who were standing outside. 'There's Darren,' we both said, and watched as Craig smiled out the window at him. It was a fleeting, anxious smile, barely seen and which never touched his eyes. We drove deep into the car park and parked up in a spot that was some distance from where the others stood. I got out of the car and took the wheelchair from the boot and assembled it beside the back door, ready for Craig. It broke my heart to see him looking out the window, and up to where Darren stood. The expression on his face still haunts me to this day. I opened the door and Craig looked at the wheelchair and then over my shoulder to Darren in the distance. He looked so sad; so very, very sad. I lifted him from the car and placed him into the wheelchair and the whole time I watched as Craig looked past me and up to where Darren stood.

I turned to Barbara and we both felt it. We felt his pain. It smothered us. We couldn't bear to see him so sad. Darren's presence had always lit a fire under Craig. He was always so excited to see him, to spend time with him. But this time it was very different. I think for Barbara and for me this was almost too much to take. We had been relying on Darren's visit to elevate Craig, to bring him happiness and rejuvenate him. When Craig looked so sad we felt defeated. It was as if something of Craig's spirit had been broken and we had just then realised it couldn't be fixed . . . but then Darren stepped in—and changed everything.

We walked up towards the others, wheeling Craig in his chair, and feeling such heaviness in our hearts. Darren walked down a little to meet us and looking at his nephew said 'Howya, Craig.'

'Hi, Darren,' was all that Craig could offer. He looked up at his uncle and his anxiety could not be disguised. Darren started to small talk with him as we all walked into the hotel lobby and found a cluster of seats to claim for ourselves. I lifted Craig from his wheelchair into one of the more comfortable seats before we all settled in. There was a distinctly awkward and horrible atmosphere in those first few moments. It was a mood of defeat and of terrible sadness. But that's when Dar came into his own.

Barbara had just left her seat to visit the bathroom and so, seeing the opportunity, Dar moved over to her vacant place beside Craig and spoke with him. He produced a packet of horror Top-Trump cards and handed them to him. Craig smiled. He spoke with Craig as he'd always done and Craig responded. He made jokes and teased him a little. Within moments Craig had been prised out from the shell where he'd hidden and emerged as the spirited, witty and life-loving Craig that we all knew. It was as though heavy chains had been stripped away from him and he was now free to be himself. From *that* moment the day was transformed. We ended up staying there for hours. We enjoyed endless laughter and a lightness of heart that we'd all needed so desperately— none more so than Craig. It was just wonderful.

It was so uplifting and heart-warming to see Craig happy again. It was so refreshing to see the strength of his character come through once more and to enjoy the majesty of his wit. At one point Craig had us all in stitches with his particular turn of phrase. He had just fallen out of his chair while excitedly playing with Darren and we'd had to lift him back up into it. He was laughing the whole time and wasn't hurt at all; far from it in fact. A few moments afterwards, Darren quizzed Craig about what had just happened, something along the lines of 'What were you doing there?'

Craig just looked at Darren and said, 'Falling out of my chair!'

We all laughed. It was so perfectly witty and so quick. But then Darren continued, 'No, I mean what were you doing after that?'

'Getting back up!' he chuckled.

Well, we all burst into laughter again at the speed of his retort. It was honest, accurate and so wonderfully quick-witted. It was just a great moment and it so perfectly captured Craig's strong personality. At that point we knew Craig had forgotten his illness, or at least it didn't seem to matter to him. He was back to being himself. His spirit had been lifted, and he had lifted ours. We soared together and drifted blissfully upon the easy currents.

It was such a beautiful thing—to spend an afternoon with Craig as he laughed and smiled throughout; to witness the peace and the serenity in his face—a face that would have you believe otherwise—as he enjoyed hour upon hour of fun. He was just a six-year-old boy and this is what he should have been doing all along. In the preceding weeks, fun had become something unfamiliar to Craig. He had slowly begun to weaken and buckle under the onslaught of his cruel illness. The little he had left was taken from him with the passing of each day. He grew sicker, weaker and more troubled as the days slipped by. Watching Craig in the hotel that day gave Barbara and me such a warm feeling. We were so happy to see him with joy in his heart, to see him giggle. We were so thankful that Dar had come over and that he'd given Craig this wonderful gift of being himself again. It was priceless and eternal and entirely unforgettable for all of us there who witnessed it.

At one telling moment during that day I lifted Craig onto my back and brought him to the toilet. In my ear Craig asked a question:

'Daddy, where is Darren sleeping tonight?'

'I don't know, Craig,' I answered. 'He never said.'

'Oh . . .' Craig said, sounding a little worried.

'I'm sure he'd love to stay down in Gorey with you, though,' I continued. 'Will I ask him?'

'YEEAAaahh DO!' Craig came alive with excitement.

In the toilet we spoke about how much fun we were having. He was just so happy. When he was ready I hoisted him back up onto my shoulders and we made our way out. Just before we came through the last door and back out into the hotel lobby, Craig spoke again into my ear, 'Don't forget to ask Darren!!'

But if that didn't tell me just how much Craig wanted to spend more time with his uncle, what came later certainly did. I had already asked Dar to come to Gorey and he'd jumped at the chance. Later on I brought Craig to the loo again and when we were in there Craig asked, 'Daddy, is Darren REALLY coming down?'

It was clear how much Craig wanted it to happen. He was actually worried that it mightn't come true. I looked Craig right in the eye and told him, 'Oh yes, he's definitely coming down.'

'BRILLIANT!'

Towards the end of the day we contemplated spending Christmas up in Lynhams. We envisaged having the same fantastic experience again, snug in the warmth and comfort of this beautifully placed hotel. But more than that, it was the power of planning ahead and seeing

Craig being strong and happy there with us all. It was comforting to think of us all being there at that time. My mother even approached the desk and enquired about hotel rooms around the Christmas period. It felt right. But we had enjoyed ourselves so much that day that leaving it until Christmas seemed just too long to wait. So before we left we decided that we would come back on the Saturday, only two days away. We wanted to recreate the perfect day that we'd just had. We wanted more of the same. We wanted to see Craig being so happy again.

Darren, as promised, joined us in the car as we headed to Gorey, with my parents returning home to Bray. It was actually quite late when we got home that night. We had spent the best part of the day, and night, up there in Lynhams and we were all quite tired when we got home. When we came in, though, Craig was quick to make sure that Darren sat with him on the couch—not that Darren had any objections, mind you. Craig took out his Yu-gi-oh cards and Top-Trumps and started to play a few games with his uncle. They sat there trading cards, just laughing and messing around. It was all so easy and so comfortable and so full of promise. Hearing Craig laughing like that continued to be such sweet music to our ears and it was the perfect note on which to end that perfect day.

The following morning we decided to travel up to Liffey Valley shopping centre. We were going to see the film *Open Season* and were delighted that Craig actually wanted to go. Before, he hadn't wanted to because he was worried about getting sick in the cinema. But this time he was ok. When we got there Darren pushed Craig in his wheelchair as we made straight for the cinema. Barbara came with us as we bought the tickets and ordered our popcorn and sweets, but wouldn't be joining us for the film. She was going to have a look around the shops and leave the 'three lads' to do our thing. She placed Craig's popcorn on his lap and gave him a kiss, saying she'd see us all later. She was just about to leave when Craig's grip faltered on the popcorn, sending the box to the ground and the popcorn all over the place. Craig looked embarrassed and my heart sank for him. There were lots of people around and he didn't need that extra attention. It was bad enough for him that he was in the wheelchair. I reached over and picked up the box which was now only half full. 'Don't worry about it, Craig!' we all seemed to say at the same time. 'It's fine, these things happen!' I placed the box back on his lap and for a moment wasn't sure what next to do. I don't know why, I think I just wanted to pretend as if nothing had happened and just go straight into the cinema. There was still plenty of popcorn in the box and Darren and I had enough to go around anyway. But I was so thankful and proud for what Barbara did in that moment. She instantly, without any hesitation, walked up to the teller and asked for a whole new box of popcorn. They had seen what happened and filled the box accordingly. Barbara came over and gave Craig the *full* box that was rightfully his, and I watched as he smiled up at her. He was so much happier and that smile said so much. He loved his mammy for doing that for him.

Inside in the cinema we parked Craig's wheelchair near the screen and I lifted him out, carrying him up to the better seats higher up near the back. Darren and I sat on either side of him as he happily munched away at the popcorn. In the distance, far below us, the wheelchair and everything it represented sat half-lit in the dim, reflected light. I hated it.

During the film all three of us laughed at some of the funnier scenes . . . and how good it was to hear Craig's giggles and unrestrained laughter. I thought of how the darkness perhaps offered Craig some sort of shelter. *Did he feel safer, more anonymous, less visible here? Maybe.* My mind raced back to the restaurant in Wexford Town where Barbara and Craig and myself had eaten food one day—Craig had become quiet and sullen, looking down at his plate and appearing awkward. We asked him what was wrong and he told us. He looked across at me and over my shoulder to the table behind where the children were staring at him; at his face. Craig's personality had been momentarily imprisoned by the skin of his disease. Sitting in the cinema, between Darren and me, Craig was free.

During the quieter moments of the film I could hear Craig chomping away. I'd occasionally glance over to my right and watch him. His face, that beautiful face of his, shimmering as if in moonlight and lost in the reprieve that this film provided. I looked at him and my heart filled with such sorrow; for the pain and torment he was suffering and yet he was just a boy. I watched as he struggled with the popcorn—his contorted arm clumsily steadying the paper bucket, while the other freely shoved fistfuls into his mouth. I smiled though as I saw how happy he was. At one point I must have been staring too long. Craig looked right at me and one half of his brow furrowed, *What?* I took the hint and looked away, smiling. But always, there under my nose, was that bloody wheelchair grounding me back into the bitter reality.

After the movie we met up with Barbara and headed to the food court to have some grub. We grabbed a seat and got Craig some McDonald's food. Darren and I quickly headed to BB's to get two coffees, but when we came back Craig was very distant with me. He was angry. It pained me to see him like that. I believe he was angry because Darren and I had gone for that coffee, and that he wasn't able to come running after us. He was frustrated at being trapped like that. He would have come running over and just stood with us. Maybe he blamed me for not even asking him to come with us. I don't know. All I do know is that his anger stemmed from a realisation of his predicament, of the liberties denied him, and he was hurting.

——

Darren stayed with us again that night and the following day we were all set to go back to Lynhams. The morning began well, with Craig in seemingly great spirits. He was lying out on the double bed while Barbara was near the window dressing table. As he lay there, and without warning he turned to his mammy and said, 'I'm going to dream of boobs, money and champagne.'

Barbara laughed out loud. What wonderful words; what zest for life, what spirit.

Later that morning Dar and I went up to Joanne's coffee shop to get some food for lunch while Barbara stayed at home with Craig. It was only while we were gone that Craig revealed he was tired. He told his mammy that he wasn't feeling too good, that he had a headache, but when she said that we didn't have to go Lynhams that day Craig was insistent that we go. When Dar and I returned Barbara told me what Craig had said—she didn't think he was able.

Craig was lying out on the sofa and looked tired, exhausted in fact. I came in on my own to him and sat beside him on the couch. I told him I had something to ask him and I hoped that he wouldn't mind. He looked at me and I simply said, 'Is it ok if we don't go to Lynhams today? . . . I'll go if you really want to go but to be honest I'm not really up to it today. What do you think?'

Craig smiled up at me and just said, 'I'm not in the mood either,' with a look of relief falling across his face.

'Let's just stay here and relax in front of the TV all day, will we?' I continued.

'Yeah,' Craig sighed, smiling yet again as the notion of the quieter day ahead soaked in.

That evening Dar knew that he had to head back to Bray and leave his little sidekick behind. Craig and Dar had been inseparable for the three days they spent together and so he knew his departure would not be welcomed as such. Barbara and I had watched Craig become revitalised for those few days and so we were anxious about Dar leaving. *How would Craig respond?*

As soon as Craig realised what was going on he was saddened. He didn't want his Uncle Darren to go anywhere and that was that. Seeing this, Dar had an idea. While nobody else was in the room and Craig was lying out on the sofa, and looking glum, he walked over to the back of the couch and whispered in Craig's ear.

'Listen, Craig, don't tell anybody, but the reason I have to go back to Bray is that I've been wearing the same underpants for the last few days and they're all shitty—I need to change them!' Darren cupped his hand to Craig's ear as he sought to emphasise the secrecy.

Craig loved it. It was pure fodder for mischief and so without a moment's hesitation he called out—'Maaammy! . . . Darren has shitty underpants!'

'Oihh!' Darren interrupted as he exaggerated his concern, but was delighted to see Craig being upbeat and mischievous again. *Result!*

It had worked a treat. Craig was giggling, the mood was lifted and Darren left without any of the trauma that only moments before looked likely. What Darren didn't know, however, what none of us knew, was that those words were to be the last he'd ever hear from Craig again.

————

The next morning, Sunday morning, Craig was violently sick. He was screaming with the pain in his head—the morphine just not doing its job. We rang the Call Doc who arrived within no time and who administered morphine intravenously. He told us that Craig shouldn't be in that type of pain and that his morphine dosage needed to be changed if it was not adequate.

Craig slept on the sofa soon after the morphine was given, leaving Barbara and me to stand over him, absorbing the grim picture before us. We were of course relieved to see Craig free from the screaming pain but still a greater fear weighed heavily down upon us. We felt so bloody helpless.

We decided it would be a good idea to bring Craig's bed down from his room and set it up in the sitting room to give him more comfort. The couch was no longer adequate for him, for his needs, and we wanted him to be as comfortable as possible. So while he slept we put it in place in the corner of the room and transferred him across.

Craig stayed in his bed and although his headache was gone he continued to vomit throughout the day. The sickness was just terrible for him. What he had to endure was unthinkable. We witnessed him being dragged through hell and yet, inconceivably, he didn't really complain. He'd get sick over and over again and then just carry on.

I remember that evening we were sitting in the front room watching TV when Craig, who was lying out on his bed, turned to me and asked would I bring him to the toilet.

'Of course, Spud,' I said, before lifting him up and out to the downstairs toilet in the hall. In the toilet I balanced Craig in a half standing position, taking his weight with my shoulder as I pulled down his trousers and then lifted him onto the toilet seat. He was very weak at this stage. His energy levels were very low and he was most likely in a permanent state of pain that he probably never really told us about. The result meant he wasn't even able to hold himself upright on the toilet, so, crouching down I had to lean into him while he rested his head on my right shoulder. We sat in that position for a while, talking about different things, as Craig waited for things to move. The warmth of his head and the softness of his skin, as he rested into the curve of my neck, filled me with such a powerful sense of love. I had my arms around him hugging his body and holding it tight. Too tightly perhaps, for my heart was broken. The reality that it had come to this terrified me. I wanted to hold him and protect him from all the evil that was bent upon him but knew that I was powerless against it.

There was silence for a moment as I could hear Craig's breathing labour slightly under the pressure of trying to push; even this small task demanded so much of him. The silence was broken then with words that I will never, ever forget. Craig gathered his breath inward and then simply whispered into my ear, 'Daddy . . . I'm going to kill this lump no matter what.' I wasn't prepared for it. Craig hadn't spoken of his illness in that way for some time. My shoulders shuddered, my lips thinned and my chin shook as I fought to suppress the waves of emotion from within. My eyes welled up and I hugged Craig even tighter. I would not let Craig see me cry. *I won't let it happen*, I thought. I pushed it downwards and exhaled it out. In a still voice I replied, 'I know you will, Craig!' as I gripped his shoulder firmly, affirming my belief in him. 'I know you will, darlin' . . . you're the master of your body, not that silly lump.'

We stayed there in the safe silence for a moment, our heads touching but facing in opposite directions. Tears streamed down my face. I'd never felt such intense and intoxicating pride as I did in that moment. And I'd never felt so utterly devastated, helpless and incredibly scared. I listened as Craig breathed heavily through his nose and mouth while surrendering the weight of his head more and more to my shoulder. He was only six and he was exhausted, but he was fighting it all the way. For all the things which that evil cancer stole from him, it couldn't touch his spirit. I was in awe at the might of him.

Then Craig said something else in my ear—'Can you smell my poo?' the faintest exhausted giggle escaping wearily from his mouth, knowing that my head was right over the bowl. *What an indomitable spirit.*

––––

We have always known Craig to be an outstanding person. There are many occasions throughout his life where we've borne witness to his remarkable shows of character strength. We've always been filled with the highest admiration for just how determinedly he pursued all those things that mattered to him, whether they be trivial or of the highest importance to him. I have never known anyone in my lifetime who has shown such strength in the face of crippling adversity like Craig did. I have never been so overwhelmingly proud and so utterly devastated in the same moment as when I think back on these difficult and powerful moments in Craig's life.

Craig at that moment was violently ill. He was disfigured, unable to walk and his left arm had become permanently contorted into a closed, locked position. It was extremely distressing for us to watch him in this state. He was shrivelling before our very eyes and it terrified us to think of what may (what would) come next. We lived with the pain of *watching* our son diminish each day, while he had to *endure* it.

He never spoke much about what was happening to him either. When things started to go wrong he merely accepted it as normal and kept doing whatever he was going to do. I remember even when his arm had first begun to lose its power and co-ordination how he'd never said a thing. We had only casually noticed how things were becoming more difficult for him to hold and had asked him about it. It was only then that he said his arm had been feeling kind of funny for a while and that it just wasn't the same as it used to be. But that was Craig all over. He always carried on, making no big to-do about it, preferring to just get on with things. He didn't like the fuss. But here we were now, at a stage where Craig was completely incapacitated by his deteriorating condition and with us having to carry him everywhere around the house.

———

The next morning Craig was desperately sick. We had to increase his morphine dosage again and arranged for Anne to call out to see him. But the very worst moment was to follow. Craig tried to talk to us, to ask us something, and we just couldn't understand him. He looked at us with growing frustration and cried out the words to make them louder, but it was no use. His tongue, his ability to form words was gone. All that we could hear were changing noises. The more he tried the angrier he got, until eventually the frustration in his eyes was replaced with something far worse—fear.

He looked out at us and knew that we couldn't understand him. Though we tried to hide it he could no doubt see the terror every bit as much in our eyes as we saw in his. That look that Craig gave us, realising his situation, was one of such exquisite pain and terror that when we reflect upon it now it threatens to undermine the very stability of our minds. His eyes, the fear in them, revealed what his lips could not. He looked to me; he looked to his mammy; and then he looked away. *He was alone.* Alone in a way that he'd never known. He was trapped inside a physical prison, looking out with one eye.

His physicality had diminished so rapidly that even confined to the bed he could no longer turn himself over. We would talk to him, asking questions requiring only yes/no answers. We would talk too much; ask too much; move his position too much, too little. We didn't know what we were doing. And all the time Craig would lie there, looking so depressed.

The hardest thing for me personally was that Craig had become so angry with me. When I spoke he didn't want to listen. When I tried to move him or touch him, he'd flinch. All I wanted to do was climb in beside him, hug him and tell him that I was going to make it all go away, but I couldn't. I had said that before. I had promised him that all along. But I had failed; broken that promise. Now Craig was looking at me with eyes that were filled with anger. But I took it. If he needed to purge himself of the fear and anger that was clearly writhing within him then I'd be that punch bag for him. I tried not to see it personally, but I knew it was there: that I had surely failed him in the worst way and he knew it.

At one point I spoke to Craig, leaning over him at his bedside, just asking him was he ok, when he turned and looked right at me. He couldn't say anything but I watched as his right arm emerged from underneath his pillow and, shaking uncontrollably while rising into the air, gave me the two fingers. I smiled, though. I knew there was humour in that gesture. He was saying that he was angry with me, but in front of all who watched in the room he played to the audience. Of course there was so much hurt there, but Craig—even then—sought to lighten the mood, his incredible personality always shining through.

When Anne arrived that morning she fitted Craig with a morphine pump which automatically administered the necessary levels into his system via an intravenous connection to his stomach. This was yet another crushing blow for us. Despite its necessity and the relief it offered it was but another of the many grim elements that had so rapidly convened around our little boy and that marked out a most unthinkable path for him.

But it did bring some measure of comfort to Craig. He no longer got sick or complained of blistering headaches, that was for sure. But those pains were replaced by listlessness, fear and a sadness that stole your breath to look upon. He was being buried alive before our very eyes, under a failing body and behind an impenetrable wall of silence. He lay there, just listening—enduring. His eyes looked out, expressing thoughts that we could never hear. Friends and family were calling in and spending time with him; holding his hand as he watched and listened to their words. They'd sit with him and then go. I'd watch, but my heart was torn by the slow realisation: *They were saying goodbye.* I'd observe their sentiment but all the while I cried out for them to hold on and not give up on him. Even then, in the face of such a precipitous fall I hung on. *How could I not?* I wanted people to rally together and believe that Craig could do it. But people were saying their goodbyes. I wondered if Craig knew this. I was terrified that those eyes, those sad and frightened eyes of his, knew.

The following day was Halloween. It was a day that would ordinarily see Craig so excited—but not this time. We awoke that morning and brought Craig back down to his bed but he was clearly very low. We got him comfortable and put the TV on but he was so distant. The most painful thing was to watch how he just reached down and, struggling, managed to pull the blanket over his face. No matter what we tried he just kept pulling that blanket over his face, lying still and hidden from us and the world. As I write this now the pain surges once again. I just cannot explain the torture of seeing your son in that state. We scratched our heads and rubbed our necks in complete frustration and overwhelming despair. *What can we do for him? How do we make this better?*

Craig's movements had diminished further and the morphine was making him sleep a lot. Barbara decided that she needed to know where this was leading. She wanted to know what this all meant for Craig. She picked up the phone and rang Anne.

'He's only got a matter of days now,' Anne said as honestly as she was asked to be. Barbara, with tears running down her face, got off the phone and told me. I was floored. I wasn't expecting to hear those words and their utterance brought me to my knees. I shook my head and wept. We held each other and cried relentlessly, squeezing each other tightly as we stood in the hall, drowning in the horror of our reality. We made our way into the sitting room and stood over our beautiful, sleeping boy. We looked down upon his beautiful face and begged whatever supposed God there was to please save him.

Halloween day came. We were dreading the constant interruptions at the door during the night, so to avoid this we decided to disconnect the doorbell and placed a sign on the front door asking people to not trick or treat as there was a very sick child within. This worked—during that whole night there came not one knock upon that door. We heard kiddies giggling and shuffling by outside but none disturbed us.

Earlier that day a friend and former neighbour of ours, Lavinia MacNeill, called round with a bag of assorted treats for Craig. They were to be the only sweets he would get for that, his last ever Halloween. We were glad that he at least got something and that the holiday hadn't completely forgotten him.

Our families had left us early that day and so we spent that Halloween evening just sitting on the sofa, glimpsing at the TV as Craig remained unconscious on the other side of the room. We sat there with our stomachs sick with fear and our hearts yearning for Craig's miracle to come. We privately thought of all the kids who were having parties or sleepovers, laughing and screaming together and having fun while our little boy lay sick in his bed. We wrestled with those demons as the night began to slip away and with it all chance of Craig experiencing it. But then at almost exactly 11 p.m. Craig stirred over in his bed. He twisted and turned his head to look over at us. In a movement that came so quick and was so unexpected he thrust his body upwards and managed to sit up. Barbara and I were stunned and before we almost had the chance to react he went to launch himself off the bed. But we got to him just in time. We held his arms as, in a fit of frustration and absolute determination, he willed himself to walk across the floor. His legs, though powerful, had no co-ordination or flexibility to do his bidding. We could feel the anger in Craig's arms as he fought us off from holding him, wanting desperately to take control once more and not succumb to that which sought to destroy him. Our hearts raced at this extraordinary show of responsiveness and awareness. We were lifted by Craig's strength, his firmness of purpose and his resolve to overcome. The three of us eventually ambled over to the couch with Craig sitting beside his mammy and leaning his back into her. I was alive with feelings of hope and of admiration for what I'd just witnessed. *He's beating this*, I thought. *He's turning a corner.*

We asked him was he hungry and he nodded yes. *Brilliant.* We asked him did he want some toast and again he nodded yes. *He's getting his appetite back.* I ran out and made some toast, feeling so elated, and then brought it into Barbara to feed him. She took a small bite of the toast and placed it in his mouth. But as we watched Craig's mouth did little. We watched as no chewing movements or tongue actions of any kind occurred. Craig's eyes began to water and he looked at us. *He couldn't swallow.*

'Can you not swallow it, darlin'?' Barbara asked, as Craig just stared into the distance. She reached her finger in and pulled the small bit of toast from his mouth as Craig looked on with tear-filled eyes. Barbara and I glanced at each other and we knew. The imponderable agony of that moment is something that neither of us can ever forget. In that moment I knew. I knew that Craig wasn't getting better; that he was slipping away; that he could no longer eat or drink and as such was showing the final symptom as explained by the consultant in Crumlin. In that moment, as Craig cried and lay still, looking away into the nothingness, I knew he was dying and that it was the cruellest death I'd ever seen in my life. This little boy, who did nothing but love and enrich the lives of everyone he met, was being slowly tortured to death in the most inhumane fashion and I could scarcely breathe as I sat by and allowed it to happen. I was his daddy. Those beautiful blue eyes of his looked out at me—crying for me to help him—and I did nothing. He leaned back into his mammy and with glistening eyes just stared upwards. Depressed.

When he went back to his bed he pulled the blanket over his face again, hiding away from the eyes of the world.

The next day we had many of our family around again. They stayed and took turns speaking with Craig and keeping him company as before. But as the day progressed Craig became more uncomfortable. He began to writhe and wriggle slightly, kicking a leg and making a moaning noise to get our attention. We tried desperately to under-stand what it was he was telling or asking us. We would try and give him a drink with small wet sponges but that wasn't it. In the end we realised that he needed to go to the toilet. Everybody left and we stayed with him as we told him to go where he was. We reassured him that we would catch it and urged him to go. But try as he might only a small amount came.

As the day moved on Barbara and I noticed that Craig's stomach was looking slightly distended. We mentioned it to Anne and she thought it possible that his bladder was overfilling. Clearly Craig hadn't wee'd in a while. Anne asked us to watch over this and to let her know if he went naturally.

That evening, after Anne's suggestion, we also decided to let her arrange for a night nurse to stay with us. We were completely drained and were worried that Craig may have a seizure. It would be a comfort for us to know that there'd be a trained nurse with him through the night were this to happen. So that night, as we sat on the couch, the night nurse stayed with us, with Craig. He was out of it completely all evening but I still brought it to the nurse's attention about his stomach being now so exceptionally distended. As soon as she saw it she rang the call doctor to arrange for a catheter. Craig's bladder was completely bloated and desperately needed to be drained. He must have felt so uncomfortable. Unfortunately the call doctor was in Wexford and we ended up having to wait almost an hour before he arrived. But then it got worse. When he arrived he had no catheter. There had been some miscommunication between himself and the nurse, with him believing that she already had a catheter with her. The nightmare of this scenario was that regardless of who was at fault, the only catheter that was available was back down in Wexford. This meant that it would be another hour and a half before they'd have it. We were disgusted.

The nurse eventually decided to drive down and get it herself and so after another hour and a half, and with the doctor called again to administer it, we were all ready to go. We were reassured by the doctor and nurse that the heavy morphine dosage Craig was under would mean he'd never feel a thing. He was apparently almost comatosed. But we knew this tube would be run up through Craig's willy and that it was a notoriously painful procedure to have to endure so we were worried for him.

As they removed Craig's pants, Craig began to make noises under his breath. And as soon as the tube was inserted, and despite all the previous reassurances, Craig screamed his little heart out. His eyes were closed and his limbs didn't move, but he screamed with the pain. We hugged him closely, terrorised by the fact that underneath his apparent unconsciousness he was indeed aware. We were horrified at the screams of pain coming from the depths of him, when he was meant to be out of it. We held him and told him that it would be over in a second and assured him that it would take away the pain in his belly. As soon as the catheter was in place the bag began to fill with urine. There was so much. Craig's stomach returned to normal and he went quiet once again. We hoped that he was feeling the relief and that it had been worth the previous torment.

But we were scarred by those screams. The implication was that he was still perfectly conscious underneath the heavy sedation and that he was still feeling pain. This was a frightening revelation for us. Our minds questioned what was really going on.

As soon as this was done Barbara and I decided that we were taking Craig up to our bed again, with the nurse remaining downstairs and only occasionally popping in to check on him. We felt more comfortable having him up there with us. As was normal at this stage, Craig stayed in the bed with Barbara but this time I slept on the floor at the end of the bed.

The following morning we woke with the nurse popping her head in to say goodbye. I actually decided to get up at that point to do some vacuuming, just to get the place clean for when people would arrive later. When I finished this I came back up to Barbara and Craig. As I came into the room Barbara was just walking across the floor on her way to the toilet. But as she did so, the strangest thing happened. Craig actually opened his eyes and followed her across the room. We were shocked to see him awake and moving his head like that.

'I'm just going to the toilet, darling,' Barbara said as she looked at him. 'I'll be back in a second. Daddy's here.' With that she moved in to the en suite.

I looked at Craig and he looked straight back at me. And then he just closed his eyes.

'I'm here with ye, darling, ok?' I said, as I sat on the end of the bed and put my hands on his legs. But as I watched him I couldn't avoid what was happening before my eyes.

'I think he's going blue!' I shouted out to Barbara, as a distinct blueness took over the complexion of his face, especially around the mouth. Barbara came out and could see it too. I grabbed the phone and rang the doctor. We sat with Craig and watched as he struggled to get air into his lungs. His heart was pounding and his chest was expanding furiously, desperately trying to pull in oxygen.

Dr Breslin arrived very quickly, carrying with him an oxygen cylinder. He placed a mask around Craig's face and allowed the oxygen to be fully inhaled. We stood and watched but it was clear that it was having no impact on Craig's colour. In fact, Craig was getting bluer. The oxygen was simply not being absorbed. Craig's lungs were filled with too much fluid for any oxygen to have a chance of being taken in.

Anne Gortland arrived not much later. She came into the room and looked at Craig as we stood next to him. She then looked at us.

'He's going now,' she said, the words almost too imponderable to understand. 'Lie in beside him and talk to him; let him know that you're with him.'

Barbara and I crouched and surrounded Craig, holding him close and talking with him. The impossible reality was upon us and we were terrified. We held Craig and hoped that this was simply not true. But it was. Barbara knew it. I knew it. Craig was about to die in front of our eyes.

'Tell him a story,' Anne suggested, tapping me on the shoulder before leaving the room to give us privacy. Anne knew about the countless bedtime stories that I—that Craig and I—had composed together. In the supercharged emotion of that moment she had seen how beautiful it would be, how fitting, for Craig to have one final bedtime story before his long sleep.

Everything in me did not want to begin a story in that moment. It felt like I was finally giving up on Craig. But I had to let go. It was time. Craig was leaving and we, his mammy and daddy, had to help make it as comfortable for him as we could. So, holding his hand and rubbing his face I spoke . . .

———

Once upon a time there was a brave and special young boy who lived with his mammy and daddy. He loved them so much and they loved him even more. One morning the handsome little boy awoke early while his mammy and daddy were still sound asleep. It was a dark morning and it looked scary out but the little boy was not afraid. Well, he was a little afraid, but he knew he was braver still. He put on his warmest clothes and walked outside, looking at the woods before him. He had been in those woods so many times and he knew them well, but in the darkness of that morning they looked very scary. But then, without a second thought the little boy walked right in. He loved adventure and exploring and this was exciting. Onwards he moved, deeper and deeper into the woods until finally he began to worry that he was lost. He had never come this way before and he couldn't remember how he got there. Just then, a beautiful light shone through the trees, from a point not too far ahead of him. The little boy thought it was the most beautiful sight he'd ever seen and found himself, ever so slowly, walking towards it. When he got there it was the most magical and beautiful place he'd ever been in his entire life. There were other children there and he felt so safe and happy as he played and ran with them. He kept smiling and laughing as he ran here, there and everywhere, hiding and chasing and having such wonderful fun. But then the little boy had a thought and he became sad. He looked back at the dark wood from where he had come and he frowned. 'I'm lost! I can't find my way home. I miss my mammy and daddy,' he sighed.

Just then a figure stood beside him and placed a large warm hand softly on his shoulder. 'Do not worry, little boy,' he said. 'Your mammy and daddy already know where you are and they are so happy you have found this place. When they wake up they will come and find you and you will all be together again. It won't be long.'

The little boy smiled because he knew it was true. He turned away from the dark wood and began playing once more in the light, happy and so full of joy.

—

When I finished this story I told Craig that if he finds that place, a bright and happy spot, he should stay there and that his mammy and I would follow him shortly. Barbara and I hugged him close and lay beside him on the bed, rubbing his arms and face and telling him that we loved him so much.

Outside Anne and Dr Breslin were sitting at the top of the stairs. They expected Craig to pass at any minute. But Craig held on. An hour passed and still Craig fought on, his face now so blue and filled with pain. Barbara and I never moved from his side.

Downstairs both our families were arriving by the minute. Anne left, telling a family member that she had an emergency to take care of, but that she would be back in a little while and that we were to ring her immediately if for whatever reason we needed to.

With all our family downstairs we decided that it would be good for people to come up and say their last goodbyes to Craig. So, one by one, his uncles, aunts, cousins and grandparents all came in and gave him a kiss goodbye. Of all those who came up that day we probably remember my sister Michelle the most. She had just arrived from England the night before and hadn't seen Craig since the summer. When she came in she gave Craig a big kiss and then left. But as she made her way down the stairs we heard her let out an uncontrollable wail. The last time she had seen Craig he'd been running around our back garden. Seeing him crippled, blue and unconscious clearly had been a most horrifying shock.

Post had arrived while we were upstairs with Craig and it was decided to bring it up to us: it was addressed to Craig. Both were parcels. The first was a small package which contained a large packet of Yu-gi-oh cards. These were the cards that Craig had ordered from eBay about ten days previously; the ones which he and I had a disagreement on—and a €50 bet. Craig had been looking for a particular card on eBay that day and as we had scrolled through the endless offers Craig stopped on one item. It was a fifty-card set which Craig told me he was sure contained the card he was looking for. I was wholly convinced that it was not among them. I went into the details of this set and there was no mention of the card in question. I said this to Craig, but he was insistent. I tried to move on and look elsewhere on the site but Craig got so frustrated and upset that I wouldn't believe him. 'It is there, Daddy!' he eventually cried at me. I couldn't bear to see him that upset so made a deal with him. I told him that I would buy him the set, but that I was betting €50 it wasn't there. Craig instantly looked up and smiled at me. 'So I get €50 as well. That's great!' his confidence, slightly disconcerting. I have to admit that I was 100 per cent certain that the card wouldn't be there, and I didn't want to see him disappointed when it didn't arrive.

So, back on the bed we quickly broke open the pack of cards and placed them into his hands to feel. 'These are the cards you ordered from eBay, darling,' we said together, as we fanned them out and moved his fingers across them. 'I'm going to see if that card—the one you wanted—is among them all right,' I said, as I took hold of them once again. I rummaged through them speaking with Craig as I did so and updating him as I went along. I knew it wouldn't be there and was prepared to give him the €50 no matter what. I don't know why I was surprised exactly, but as I sifted through the final fifteen or so cards, there it was. I would have staked my life on that card not being there, and yet here it was in my hand. I was so happy for him. *He was right.*

'You were right as usual, Spud,' I said, holding his hand and then placing the card within. 'That's the card you told me would be there and I wouldn't listen. I should have known you'd be right. You always are. Jaysus, you have €50 too.'

Barbara then opened the second, larger parcel and inside there was a small South African rugby shirt, and a letter. The letter was from her friend Keah, who was living in South Africa, and it was addressed to Craig. Barbara read it out loud to him, then put the shirt in his hand to feel. We put all the stuff aside and then lay down next to him once again.

We lay with Craig for almost six hours as his body fought on for life. We spent those hours telling Craig over and over again how much we loved him and how much he meant to us. We rubbed him. We hugged him. We whispered to him. But as the time passed Craig's chest rattled and wheezed so badly that it was sheer torture to endure. I kept moving Craig's position, hoping to free the rattle and congestion that laboured his breathing so. But his body was so strong, it clearly wasn't giving up. Craig got bluer and bluer and his hairline was wet with sweat as his body was pushed to the very extremes of survival. Both Barbara and I thought that it was just the cruellest suffering and we couldn't stand to see it happening to our boy.

Anne arrived into the room and approached us. She could see the distress on our faces. I was beginning to lose it at this point. I felt so helpless as our boy lay dying beside us, in the most horrendous fashion.

'Is there nothing can be done?' I pleaded with Anne. 'This is horrific. He's slowly suffocating to death and we're doing nothing. An animal wouldn't be allowed to die this way!'

'What are you asking me?' Anne replied softly. 'Are you asking me to give him a final dosage?'

'No! . . . I don't know,' was all I could say honestly. The thought of my son dying was too unbearable. 'I just think this is wrong. Craig suffering like this.'

'Craig is on the highest dosage of morphine I can give him, and I can promise you that he is not suffering.' Anne was quick to try and ease our pain. Barbara and I wanted to believe this was true but we had heard Craig screaming the night before while heavily under morphine. Our minds were being torn apart.

'How will he go?' Barbara then asked Anne, as she stood up beside her. Neither of us knew what to expect. Would he have some kind of fit or would he just stop breathing, we just didn't know.

'His heart will simply stop beating and he will stop breathing,' Anne said quietly, as she made a flat gesture with her hand to illustrate the point.

Just then, right at that very moment, Craig let out a breath and we watched.

'He's not breathing!' I exclaimed, as no inhalation followed.

'Quickly, get in with him,' Anne said, as Barbara then moved quickly in beside Craig again.

We both watched for the breath that never came. The moment was surreal. The blue slipped from his face and he looked beautiful, more beautiful than we could ever remember.

'Oh Craiggg!' I cried, as I pulled him towards me, his head leaning lifelessly backwards with mouth open. *He was gone.*

'NOOOoooo!' Barbara screamed, as the horror overwhelmed her. 'Oh Craig, oh my beautiful Craig! No, God, no!'

I looked into my son's eyes and felt the weight of him in my arms. I wanted to squeeze him back to life again. I simply could not understand that he was now dead. I kept crying out his name and pulling him into me. I couldn't cope with this being real. I remember looking to the corner of the room thinking he was perhaps floating there looking down at the horrific scene unfolding before him.

Barbara was on the other side holding Craig's head, roaring and hugging him. She wailed his name over and over again, incapable of believing that he was truly gone. She kissed his face and kept saying that she loved him so much, and then crying his name repeatedly.

I pulled his heavy head into my neck and kissed him on his cheek. I thought back to what he had said to me on the toilet only days before and so whispered 'You got it in the end, Craig. You killed that lump no matter what. Just like you said,' and then roared with the hideous pain that took me, crying 'Be happy, darling . . . Be happy!'

Barbara and I lay on the bed squeezing Craig and crying our hearts out as the room filled with family. They had heard Barbara's scream from downstairs and had rushed up, knowing what it meant. They stood at the foot of the bed, witnessing the rawness of our emotion and not knowing what to say. I wanted to shout out and tell everyone to leave us alone and get out of the room. I couldn't believe that they wouldn't give us the space to have that moment with Craig. I was so angry—but my sorrow was stronger. I wasn't going to let anything take away from this moment. So I lay there just crying and hugging my little boy. They stayed only briefly, however, and then left, leaving us in peace to mourn our son. In retrospect, I'm glad they came in though. I'm glad for Craig that they were all there to see him off.

Anne had suggested that we lie with him while he was still 'warm'. Even hearing those words pierced our souls. We curled up together— just the three of us—and cried as we lay there. His body was warm and his face looked beautiful. All the pain had gone from it. It didn't feel right that he looked and felt so well—so alive. But after only a short while we could feel his legs getting cooler. It was horrific. We looked down at his face and called his name but he was gone. He was dead and there was no changing it. No going back.

Dr Breslin came in after a while and officialised Craig's death before offering his sympathies and leaving. Although the undertaker offered, we told him that we wanted to prepare Craig to be laid out ourselves. We took Craig out of his clothes and washed him down with a fresh cloth and some clean water. Barbara chose the clothes she knew he'd like and then we dressed him. His body was getting so cold and it felt so horribly wrong. But we wanted to do this for him. Barbara had always dressed Craig; always picked nice clothes for him and made sure that he was looking good. This was the last time she would get to do this for him. When he was dressed, we clasped his hands together and wrapped rosary beads around them.

In Craig's room his bed had been prepared and laid out by my sister Melanie and Barbara's mother. They had done this just after Craig had passed. Ever so gently we lifted Craig from our room and carried him into his. We laid him out on his own bed and placed him under the sheets. We stood back and looked down upon our child and we cried. He went ahead of us at 4.43 p.m. on Thursday, 2 November 2006.

LIVING ON...

Chapter 8 ∾

The Silent, Painful, Empty Nothingness

Waking up the morning after Craig had died was one of the most horrific experiences Barbara and I had to go through. It was one, among many at that time, which still haunts me. There is that brief moment, where in opening your eyes your mind is free from all thought, preoccupied only with the business of becoming conscious. But then it hits you. God, how it hit me; hit Barbara. *Craig is dead. His corpse is in the other room.* I almost needed to get sick. I grunted outwards as I began to shallow breathe and weep. I turned over on my side and cried silently to myself. *Oh Jesus Christ, my beautiful Craig is dead. Oh please, please don't let this be true. Oh help me, please I can't . . . Oh Jesus no please God no.* But there was no escaping the truth. Craig was dead. Our Craig was dead. Craig was gone, and never again would we see him, hear him, smell him, talk with him, play with him, share stories with him, walk in the woods with him, chase him, mess and fight with him, laugh with him, give out to him, listen to him, answer questions for him, or simply watch him grow to become the wonderful young man that he was sure to be, building memories and sharing happiness as we grew together as a family. All gone. All wiped out as if none of it ever mattered. A life destroyed. Lives destroyed.

But we got up. We got out of our bed and headed into Craig's room. Just walking into that room and seeing him laid out sent a thousand knives through our hearts. That terrible reality. Some of Barbara's family had stayed overnight, making sure that someone was always in the room with Craig. I can't remember who was in the room that morning as we entered, Shane and Tina I think, but all I saw was my son. My precious boy. It tore at my stomach. His eyes were only half-closed, just like when he used to sleep. It could easily have been our beautiful sleeping boy but it just wasn't. Kissing him on his soft cheek and patting his head was our morning greeting to him. Tear-filled eyes dripped onto his cold face as we whispered how much we loved him and how we were sorry, so sorry, for letting this happen. For letting him down. For breaking our promise. We hugged and we held him and we apologised. I'd never felt a corpse before. I'd seen one, but never touched. Kissing Craig and feeling the chill on his skin was so terrifyingly real. I kissed and whispered and wished him alive. I begged for his return. Some miracle . . . but I knew. Still, I pleaded.

The night before, just as we were lying in bed, we had discussed what music would be best for Craig's funeral. This was a difficult discussion, neither of us wanting to think about it—about the reality of what had happened and what was to come—but we talked. One song above all had stood out immediately for me.

You'll Be in my Heart was a song that featured in the Tarzan movie. Craig used to watch this movie a lot when he was younger. I remember many times making up a bed for him in my study (spare room) out of a folded duvet, some pillows and a covering blanket. I'd put the Tarzan DVD on my computer and he would lie on the floor, with giddy smiles, and settle to camp down and watch the movie. Sometimes I would lie on the floor with him for a while, but mostly I would play my guitar in another room. Other times I would leave him upstairs to watch it. But lying in the bed that night thinking of funeral songs, it was not those memories which made me think of it.

No. It was the memory of our trip to Disneyland. We had gone to see the Tarzan live stage show there and at the very end Craig did something that stuck with me. While everyone spilled out of the theatre, Craig grabbed our hands, and told us to sit down. 'I like this song,' was all he said. I had barely taken any notice of the music which was playing over the speakers as everyone, who ignored it too, rushed out to move onto the next Disneyland attraction. But Craig noticed it. Craig had music in his soul. It was *You'll be in my Heart* and he sat down and listened to every word. Only when it was finished did he get up and say 'Come on so . . .' Lying in the bed that night that memory shot to the front of my mind and the exquisite pain of it squeezed at my throat and pulled at my stomach. Our beautiful, beautiful Craig.

The next morning Barbara and I happened to mention this song to

Shane. I had already rung my sister Melanie to see if she could get it for me so I was hoping desperately she could. Shane, however, reacted immediately saying, 'Jesus, I think I have that album in the car,' before running downstairs and outside. He returned with a Phil Collins album and he showed it to me. The song was there. I took the bedside CD player from our room and connected it in the hall outside Craig's room and began playing the song. As soon as I heard the music playing and the first line I wept. We all wept. I looked into the room and could see Barbara crying, and Shane with a watery glaze in his eyes. I stopped the CD. I thought I was going to explode with pain. I wanted to scream with angered sorrow and guilt. But Barbara asked me to keep playing the CD, so I did. The words and sentiment were so fitting. Equally they could have been from Craig's perspective or from ours and they stirred the deepest emotions within.

When Shane left we were alone for the first time with our Craig, since he passed. We both cried. We sat at his bedside and we stared at him. We talked and we stared and we cried. It was so difficult in that moment to be anything but unbearably broken. But it's amazing how the practicalities of life encroach even on the most emotional and life-changing moments. We knew that people would be arriving so we knew we had to clean the house. Barbara's mother had done a lot of it already, but still there were things to be done. We set about getting things in order while going in and out to speak with Craig and kissing him. Barbara had mentioned how much she feared the next day— seeing Craig being 'put down into that hole and never seeing him again'—and I agreed, but not really empathising with the fear that Barbara genuinely felt. To me the worst thing had already happened. Nothing beyond what had already come to pass held any fear for me. Craig was dead, and nothing or no one could hurt me any more than I was already hurting. I understood that Barbara didn't want to see our son going into a dark hole in the ground. I did. I didn't want to see it happen either. But I certainly didn't feel as anxious as Barbara. It just didn't grip me, as it did her. Even later on that evening I overheard others saying 'God it won't be easy for them tomorrow,' or 'The worst is yet to come,' or 'Wait till this is all over, and the house is empty— that's when it'll really kick in'. I heard these comments and thought nothing of them, save for the fact they were merely the well-meaning sentiments of others. In the privacy of my own thoughts I had tears only for the present; tomorrow, the next day, the day after that were of no consequence to me.

Around afternoon the undertaker, Lar Murphy, called around. We spoke up in Craig's room. 'He looks just like he's asleep,' he commented and it was so true. *He could be just asleep.* Even then, a day after he'd died, I found myself begging for some kind of miracle—that maybe he'd wake up and begin to get better. The reality, the loss, was too much to bear. We could barely function at all. The day felt surreal, like we were outside it. Even the people we would meet during the day felt distant to us, like we were spectators in someone else's life. *If only.*

Among other things, Lar had come to take Craig's measurements for his coffin. Again another surreal situation to be faced with. 'He's above average in size for his age,' said Lar, 'so I'll have to get a larger coffin.' *Above average.* Craig was many things in his short life, but average he certainly was not. He was neither a shrinking violet, nor someone to make up numbers. He was a force of nature whose self-confidence and zest for living was truly inspiring. Oh he was a rascal at times and he could have a temper when he saw fit, but he was an absolutely joyous young man all told. In how he lived his life, he was an example to me, to Barbara and to everyone who came to know him. *Above average in life; above average in death.*

As the undertaker left, a peculiar thing happened that struck us as being odd, almost humorous—incredible as that sounds. Lar had got into his car and we were back in the house when all of a sudden Lar came racing back in to us, gesturing for us to follow him out. 'C'mon, quick, it's about to come on now,' he exclaimed as all three of us were now running towards the cab of his car. In he reached and turned up the radio, quite loud, saying 'It's the death notice I put in for Craig. Listen . . .' We remember listening and then hearing those dreadful words: **Craig Sexton of Hazelwood, Gorey. Died Nov 2nd. Funeral Mass at 2 p.m., Saturday, St Michael's Church, Gorey.**

Another confirmation. Another inescapable acknowledgement of our little boy's death. But the nature of how we came to listen to that notice is something I'd never have expected. After Lar left, Barbara and I returned to the house and we both looked at each other. We actually, amazingly, kind of laughed at the picture of us running out, blindly enthusiastic to hear the death notice of our only child in the cab of the undertaker's car. It was truly bizarre and in the most unexpected and weirdest way possible we're thankful for that.

———

In contrast to that a more hideous memory of that day also comes back to me now as I write. I was in the room speaking with Craig, holding him and telling him how much I loved him. I had been there for a while. I decided to get up for a moment and go out into another room —for what, I can't recall—but I returned within a matter of seconds. When I came into the room there was a large bluebottle flying around. Well . . . I panicked, almost crying and furious at the same time. On seeing that fly my mind was immediately filled with the image of maggots. I had to protect my boy. All my life I had never wanted to hurt a creature. Barbara used to get annoyed at how I'd try to save spiders and little insects from the sink or shower. Even one evening, when a mouse scuttled across the sitting room floor as we watched the TV, I'd spent nearly thirty minutes trying to catch him in a box so I could set him free. Barbara had even woken Craig and brought him down to see the little furry animal. Try as I might I couldn't get him safely so Barbara hit the little fecker over the head with the 'safety box' to put an end to that evening's entertainment. But I just didn't like inflicting death on anything. When I saw that bluebottle in the room, however, I was going to kill it. We'd had all the windows closed to prevent this scenario, but here it was flying menacingly around Craig's room. It felt evil. After trying to get it on a number of attempts I eventually opened the window and it flew out. I didn't want to think of what may or may not have happened in the few seconds I had been out of the room. I cleaned Craig's face and hands anyway, and cried.

At mid afternoon Father JJ called around to the house to go through the funeral arrangements. He wanted the names of people who would be partaking in the mass and some information about Craig—his hobbies, favourite toys or cartoons, music he liked etc—so that he could mention this during the mass. We told him how The Simpsons was his favourite cartoon, followed closely by Yu-Gi-Oh, and that he loved so much music that it would be difficult to single out anything in particular.

One peculiar choice was Craig's love for The Dubliners so we mentioned this to Fr JJ. It was peculiar because neither myself nor Barbara ever listened to The Dubliners at home so he hadn't learned to love it through osmosis as such. No, we'd bought a newspaper one time which had a free 'Dubliner's collection' CD with it and Barbara had played it in the car one day. She was surprised when Craig, who was sitting in the back seat, asked 'Play that song again, Mammy.' The song was 'Spanish Lady' and Craig had latched onto the lyrics straight away. It was as simple as that. From that point Craig, all by himself, developed a love for The Dubliners. It wasn't long in fact before he knew most of the lyrics and he'd sing along to each song as we drove here and there.

Barbara remembers one particular morning when she was driving him to school. As was customary, she was playing some of his music, which in this case was The Dubliners' 'Spanish Lady'. Craig was sitting in the back singing his heart out. He knew every word: '. . . Cold as a fire of ashy coal' and '. . . Down by Napper Tandies place' came loudly from the back seat. Barbara parked up the car and before she got a chance to turn off the ignition Craig called out to her saying, 'Wait . . . just let me hear this song.' Barbara told him she couldn't because she'd be late for work, but Craig persisted. 'Please, Mammy . . . just to the end of the song . . . please?' Craig's joy was infectious and Barbara was powerless against it. She sat back and listened while Craig sang through every verse until the end. 'Thanks, Mammy . . . c'mon so,' was all that he said as he finally grabbed his schoolbag and got out of the car. It was only fitting that we also chose that particular song for the funeral.

Fr JJ had given us some prayers to choose from for the funeral mass. All I could remember thinking, as I read them, was 'what utter bullshit'. We had to choose one and neither Barbara nor I wanted one of them. Every prayer paid homage to a God that allowed this to be. Every prayer had us kneeling and pouring out glory to a being that allowed a six-year-old boy to die a slow, tortured death—whose weary body was slowly crippled, subjected to relentless sickness and who was left to choke slowly and cruelly to death, while we his parents lay with him, watching. We had no time for God. We wanted to rip up those prayers and burn them for the rubbish they were. But life is full of contradictions, and so despite our deepest feelings towards them, we chose one, to be read out aloud in wonderful praise of our Lord. That day was not a day for anger or for battles. It was Craig's day. It was our farewell to our special little man and nothing would spoil it.

As the day progressed more and more people began calling to the house, offering their sympathies and condolences. I knew I had to write Craig's eulogy and get his music CD so later that night, and feeling under pressure, I told Barbara that I was going to my room to get them organised.

When I sat at the computer with that blank page in front of me, I cried through gritted teeth. I was so angry and distraught that here I was sitting, trying to put together my son's eulogy. It was just so fucking wrong. It went against nature. My son's dead body was in one room and I was in another, writing words for his funeral. Writing those words nearly destroyed me. I actually felt faint, dizzy and sick. That time, spent writing those words, was again one of the most painful experiences of my life. I wanted, at one stage, to pick up the screen and throw it out the window. I was so utterly devastated—no father should ever have to write his son's eulogy.

After I'd completed it I called Barbara to the room and tried to read it to her. As I did my throat froze up and I just started to cry. I couldn't do it. I handed it to Barbara who read it with tears streaming down her face. Watching her I cried too: a mother reading her young son's eulogy. Just so bloody wrong! The whole scene was agonising . . . and just so damn unnatural.

More and more people were arriving downstairs while others stayed in the room with Craig. Craig would have loved it actually. He would have loved all those people there, and especially seeing as they were there for him. Craig was not shy; he loved people. He was at ease in the midst, or in front, of a crowd. God when I think of the amount of times he'd stand up and belt out songs or dance. And everyone was always impressed by how he knew the words to so many songs and how he sang them so animatedly.

Once, when he was about four years old, we were down home with Barbara's folks with Craig singing a song, like he frequently did, in front of all the family. Suddenly, beside me, all I could hear was a stream of laughter: Craig's granddad, Paddy, was smiling and laughing his head off. There were tears coming in his eyes. 'It's the emphasis he puts on the words—the passion,' he laughed. 'Ah it's brilliant,' he continued, before asking Craig to sing it again. I can still see Paddy's face as he sat there watching and laughing as his grandson whipped out a cracking performance for everyone; one of so many that Craig gave over the years.

———

It was lovely to see both of Craig's teachers arrive—Miss Vaughan from his first year, and Miss O'Neill from his last year—together with Adrienne, the teacher's assistant, who gave Craig such special attention in his final months of schooling. I remember thinking a couple of things as I watched them looking down at Craig's body. I wondered what was going through their minds as they looked upon the once happy and boisterous little chap, who brought such life and sunshine to their class; that wonderful little boy who was now lying lifeless in front of their eyes. I wondered if memories were running through their minds—memories that I or Barbara would never know—of happy times with Craig. I also wondered what Craig would think, having his teachers in his house looking at him as he just lay there. These thoughts ran through my mind as I watched their stares.

Miss O'Neill spoke and shared a lovely memory with us and the others who were in the room with Craig. She told us that Craig had caused her to change the way she ran her art class. Normally she used to collect up old newspapers and just let the kids spread them over all the tables before getting on with the important business of letting their beautiful little minds be creative. Unfortunately this all changed when a little man by the name of Craig Sexton was introduced into the mix. One day she noticed that Craig was holding a particular sheet of newspaper with great interest and that he had propagated an intrigue among a small gathering of his friends who apparently felt the need to huddle around him. On closer inspection, Miss O'Neill discovered that the object of their interest was a scantily clad young lady who was smiling back at the motley crew. It appears that Craig's mind had been creative after all—just in a different way. From that moment onwards a new 'screening process' was introduced to Art proceedings.

We were so happy to hear this story. It was so Craig. I could imagine him, see him in the class with his mates all gathered round as they giddily looked down at the unexpected and welcome display.

I'm certain there are many memories like this they have of Craig and I'd love to know them. All that we do know is that Craig enjoyed school. He loved being with other kids and it made it so much easier for us to see him off to school with a smile on his face each morning. As two working parents there's always that guilt I suppose—that we weren't there enough for him. Barbara was the lucky one who got to bring him to school every morning in his first year, before rushing off to work. I wish that I had those memories. There were just a few times that I was lucky enough to bring him in that first year, and I loved it. I loved the hustle and bustle of all the kids going into school, with their chatter and excitement filling the morning air. Even then I knew how cherished those memories would be for me in the future. I felt privileged being there, holding my little boy's hand as I walked him through those gates. But I never knew just how soon that future would come, and end, nor how incredibly precious those memories now are.

———

To be honest I can't really recall everyone who came that evening but it was comforting to see them showing such respect for the little man who meant so much to us. Some who came didn't even know Craig, never having met him, but they did it for us. We look back now on all those faces that shared tears and extended sympathetic arms that night and we thank them all. Maybe now, in reflecting on that night, the true power of the support is being felt. I remember different things said, people's faces and a warmth that was shown to Barbara and to me that we'll be eternally grateful for.

A strong memory I have of that night was witnessing my father alone with Craig in the room. Just before this, Barbara's mother had told her that she was feeling sorry for him after watching him up in the room. He had been pulling at Craig as he hugged and kissed him, so much so that Craig's hands, which we'd folded together and wrapped with rosary beads, had come apart. Barbara and I had noticed beforehand that his hands kept coming free, causing us to have to readjust them, but now we understood why. When I saw my father with Craig and witnessed his raw emotion and need for tactile comfort, it was like I was outside myself looking down upon my own utter despair. Craig's loss was clearly not just our own. He meant so much to so many.

———

There's no comfort to be had by anyone in these situations, and most people know this. But it never stops people from trying, nor should it. At one point I hit a real low whilst standing in the kitchen with family and others around me. I was struggling with Craig's death, as was Barbara, but in me, without the slightest doubt was the belief that Craig was still alive somewhere else and that we would meet again. Barbara didn't have this belief and as a result was very raw and exposed to the full terror of Craig's loss. I know this because, for the briefest moment, while standing in that kitchen, the thought entered my head: *What if you're wrong? What if that's it and you'll never ever see Craig again?* I was speaking with my eldest brother David at the time and I voiced it. I began crying with such despair and sadness, the possibility being too much to bear. Seeing me like this, David grabbed me by the shoulders and, crying himself, told me that of course I'd see him again and reassured me as best he could that Craig had gone to a better place and that we would see each other in time.

I needed to believe this to keep me upright. I need to believe this always and I do. But Barbara struggles with this. Her grief is a mother's grief and in the absence of a belief in an afterlife, her path is so much harder than mine. In that brief moment where I let go of the rope, I got a glimpse into the mindset of what Barbara must live through so frequently—and it's a terrifying place. I simply could not go on if I thought that I'd never ever see my Craig again. There have been 'bad days', as Barbara and I call them, where I've doubted again, and all I could do is go to bed. Those days are days where the will to live, the sense in living, abandon me. I only get these days very rarely, but Barbara gets them more. Her doubt, her fear is stronger, and I do not envy her that one bit.

Sitting at Craig's bedside that night it suddenly hit me that Craig was to be buried the next day and that we were running out of time. This was to be the last night that Craig would spend at home with us. Instantly I wanted Craig all to myself and Barbara. I wanted everyone to leave so that we could be alone with him. I was beginning to feel tired just about then and I wanted to spend the night in the room with him. I said this to Barbara and she felt the same.

With that everyone began to leave. We thanked them and soon we were on our own with Craig. We spoke with him and hugged him, rubbing his forehead and cupping his cheeks. *So cold, so bloody cold.* We got some duvets and blankets and made up a bed on the floor beside his bed. We snuggled up on the floor and spoke for a little while, but our weariness and our sadness got the better of us and we fell asleep. I think my last thought was that Craig would have loved to squeeze in between us there, on the floor . . . and Christ how we would have loved it too. We both slept fitfully that night but the morning was still too soon in coming.

––––

When we woke we went straight over to Craig. We kissed him and held him and as tears fell we silently knew the terror of what lay ahead of us that day: the terror which really only hit me the night before. It was knowing that our little boy would be leaving us forever and that we'd never see him again. I knew when he died that he was gone. But having his body with us still, being able to hug and hold him and keep talking to him, somehow masked the full truth of his absence. As people, we are creatures of touch, and as parents we express our love to our young children in a very tactile manner. So while we could still feel and hold Craig, it allowed us to continue that expression.

That morning, the thought that he would be gone from us was unbearable. I watched as Barbara placed her lips on Craig's and kissed her little boy. I stood with tears in my eyes as I watched her press a warm cheek against his cold one, closing her eyes as she dreamed away this nightmare and remembered better times. I could see the pain in her face as no arms reached up around her neck, as they so often had. I felt it all.

We readied ourselves that morning in preparation for the funeral. We washed and got dressed as quickly as we could, giving ourselves as much time with our Craig as we could. Every last second was so precious, and it was slipping away. I placed €100 into Craig's pocket.

This was made up of the €50 that I owed him from losing the bet about the Yu-Gi-Oh card and €50 that his granddan would have given him on that Friday, as he'd always done in those last few months. I kept talking to him and told him what the money was for as I placed it into his little pocket. Barbara stood at the other side of the bed and kept speaking to him, telling him that the money was his to spend as he wished.

But it wasn't long before the undertaker arrived and asked us whether we were ready to have him placed into his coffin. *The moment had arrived.* We nodded, and so he asked us to leave the room while he made the transferral. We moved to the room next door and held each other as we listened to the tussles and movement coming from Craig's room. Neither of us wanted to picture the indignity of what was going on in there, but we knew. After only a short while we were allowed back in to see him laid out in the white coffin. What a horrific sight: another step closer to the grave . . . and away from home.

We spent some final moments alone with him in the room and placed a number of special items in the coffin with him. I put a silver ring in his pocket—a ring that I sometimes wore and that Craig told me he wanted when he was older. (It had an unusual pattern that was reminiscent of the ring in *Lord of the Rings* and which appealed to Craig so much. So often when we were down in Wexford, and while Barbara was in the Villa shop, we'd wait outside looking in the window of a shop—Wexford Silversmiths, I think. It was an unusual jeweller's, with the window display housing the figure of a crouching hobbit with his hand and palm outstretched revealing a single plain gold ring. Craig was intrigued by it and always looked in.) Placing the ring in his pocket I knew I should have given it to him while he was alive: he'd obviously wanted it more than I did—the amount of times I'd found it in his room or inside the treasure box his Nana had given him!

I also put a torch into the coffin; one that straps around the head— so he wouldn't be in the dark and could find his way.

Barbara placed his Christening blanket in with him and the medal of bravery that he received from St Luke's Hospital. There was certainly no doubt about his bravery. He actually got two of those bravery medals, and we still have the second one in his room. If anyone earned those medals, a thousand of those medals, it was Craig. Barbara's sister Tina gave us a card from her kids—Jennifer, Niall,

Áine, Peter, Pádraig, Niamh and Colm—while my brother David gave us cards from his: Megan, Lauren and Sam. We placed these cards alongside Craig and told him who they were from.

Too soon we were told that it was time to go. The hearse was waiting. We kissed and held Craig and said our painful final goodbyes to our dear little boy. We desperately clambered our hands over his head and body and kept kissing and talking to him, fighting the inevitable. Every touch, every kiss, every hug was to be our last and we didn't want it to be. Finally we had to let go.

The coffin—our Craig—was finally placed in the back of the hearse. Barbara and I had our eyes fixed on that coffin as we stood outside. We were aware that there was a large gathering outside, but neither of us could take it in. As we moved, and we followed, we could only stare at the photo of Craig that rested in the back of the hearse. It was a photo of Craig in his school uniform and he had the most beautiful smile, blue eyes and dimples. With every step we took between the house and the church, we just kept watching that picture. We wished in our deepest being that this was not happening, that this was some nightmare. Our bodies were weak with despair and staring at that beautiful dimpled smile, knowing that we'd never see it again— NEVER see Craig again—was an impossible truth to accept. When we entered the church grounds there was a guard of honour made up of schoolgirls from Craig's Loreto school. I could only make this out in my peripheral vision at first, but it caused me to look briefly away from the picture. 'How's about that, Craig, eh? . . . all those girls there for you,' I thought, and in that moment as I stared back at the picture of Craig, I almost hoped to see Craig winking back at me.

Sitting at the front of the church we waited. The first song played was 'Little Willow', a song by Paul McCartney that I used to play on my guitar and which Craig used to sing along to. He loved sad songs. He was so emotionally attuned in that regard. He used to know when songs were sad and then ask me about them. I remember telling Craig about that particular song, and how the man who wrote it had done so for the children of a close family friend who had died. When that song played in the church I buckled. I could see Craig in the room with me, singing 'Bend little willow, winds gonna blow you, hard and cold tonight.' I held Barbara tight as we fell apart with tears and leaned into each other, desperate in our pain.

'Spanish Lady' was the second song played and again this hit us hard. Especially for Barbara who remembered those school trips and her backseat singer who loved to belt out that tune at the start of each day.

Neither Barbara nor I were fit to say anything at that mass, as much as we so dearly wanted to. I knew my throat would freeze and nothing would come out so we decided to ask Hugh Dunne, Barbara's brother-in-law, to read Craig's eulogy for us. When he read it out at the funeral mass, Barbara and I were inconsolable. You'll Be in my Heart began playing immediately after and it stirred so much emotion within us—memories of our trip to Disneyland, of Craig in the camp-bed in my study when he was younger. We just trembled and held each other as tight as we could.

The last song that was played was Time of your life by Green Day. Craig liked this song, and it was played as we carried Craig back out to the hearse. As that music played and I carried my child up that aisle, the pain in my heart was intolerable. I wanted to run off with him and not have to bury him in the cold darkness, which I knew was only moments away. Everything in my body screamed to not let this happen, but I knew it had to be done. That song, when I hear it now, sometimes haunts me. It is the one song that reminds me most of his death and his funeral, the others being more evocative of happier times.

As we walked out of the church, following the hearse, and making our way to the graveyard an incident occurred that will forever stay with me. The graveyard was located in a different part of the town to where the church was, so it meant that we had a bit of a walk. This didn't matter. Well, not to most anyway. For two people, it became evident this route was a little bothersome and inconvenient. I could hear them behind me somewhere, walking out of step with everyone else, and talking loudly enough to be heard and asking how much further was there to go? (I now know this was said in a more humorous context, but I didn't see it that way at first.)

My first thought was 'I can't believe what I'm hearing'. As I looked at Craig's picture in the back of the hearse I noticed that I could see the two people in question in the reflection of the hearse's back door window. I stared at their reflections for a second and before I even got the chance to lose it I found myself smiling. Miraculously I watched a rogue wasp come out of nowhere and attack the two reflections. I smiled as I witnessed flailing arms and ducking heads. I looked back at Craig's picture and winked at him, silently saying to him 'Good man, you put a stop to that.' It was very much Craig's style.

It also instantly brought to mind the day Craig had frightened the life out of a checkout girl in Pettit's with a plastic spider. He had waited until his mammy had put the last of the shopping on the conveyor belt before strategically placing an up-until-then concealed large, black, rubber spider. The first I knew of it was when I jumped—I had heard a very loud, high-pitched scream coming from the checkout woman. I had no idea what had just happened. I was packing the shopping away when the shriek of terror happened. 'Jaysus Christ . . .' she continued, now giggling (no doubt relieved) as she looked at Craig's smiling face. He was half laughing, his eyes darting between his mammy, me and his victim—his pure exhilaration tempered only by the fact that he was momentarily unsure as to whether he was going to be in trouble or not.

So seeing that timely wasp playing with its deserved victims had Craig written all over it. When I look back now I'm so glad that little incident happened. It was at once an unexpected moment of disbelief, of humour and of intense beautiful connection with Craig—a moment we're so deeply thankful for.

Arriving at the graveyard we had no clue where we were going. When the hearse finally rested at the top of the graveyard we looked over and both could see the spot. The imminent terror was upon us. Barbara was overcome with emotion at this point and it took everything in my power to hold myself together. When it came to lowering Craig into that deep, deep hole I could barely think straight. I had even grabbed one of the lowering ropes at random until Barbara's brother Shane came over and asked me did I want to take the rope nearest the head. I'm glad he did. Looking down as Craig's body descended into that earth was terrifying. Feeling his weight in my hands and imagining, beyond the lid, his face looking back up at me was just horrific.

I went over to Barbara then and held her in my arms as she cried desperately for her little boy. I hugged her close—for her and for me. Were I there on my own, facing the nightmare alone, I fear I would have crumbled under the unbearable grief. But we had each other to lean on. Neither I nor Barbara can remember how many people were there. Neither of us ever looked up to see. We were fixed on that piece of ground and our little boy. But there were many, so we're told.

We stayed there at his graveside for a while; until most people left. My brother Dave had his car nearby and offered us a lift back to the house but we chose instead to walk it quietly together. We knew that we weren't up to speaking with people. On the way up through the estate we passed a dog that we were familiar with. He was a cocker spaniel, I think, and he always lay outside on the front lawn of his house. He was the most docile dog you could hope to meet. He was the type of dog you could nearly walk over and he still wouldn't budge. This time, however, as we passed by he was sitting upright and as we approached he raised his paw and made some yelping noises at us. We both kept walking but thought it extremely odd. (I suppose it's funny really, but a couple of days afterwards I was walking home from the graveyard when I happened to be passing that dog again. It was kind of dark but oddly again he was sitting upright, looking at me. I got a bit emotional and began approaching the dog as if there was something profound going on—as though he was sympathising with me. But that was bollocks . . . he went for me! All teeth and growls coming at me as I hop skipped my arse out of there. When I reached a safe distance I had a little laugh to myself.)

When we got back to the house we headed straight to our bed, too depressed to see or speak with anyone. We held each other and we cried. We talked. We listened to the voices of many people downstairs. We even felt like we were being terrible hosts. Ridiculous, isn't it. Barbara's mother came up to bring us a cup of tea and some toast and then left us be. I'm not sure how long we stayed there in that bed but we did eventually decide to get up and go downstairs. I ended up sitting in the kitchen with some family and friends of mine and Barbara stayed in the sitting room with hers. We were poor company but that didn't matter. It certainly didn't matter to me. We chatted as best we could and it was quite late before everyone had gone. With the house empty we headed to our bed and tried to sleep. But sleeping wasn't the problem; it was the waking which proved so painful.

The avalanche of reality and sorrow which descends so rapidly on you is overwhelming. In the cold light of the morning, with not a sound in the house, the feeling of absolute despair is acute. You cry and beg for it all to be untrue. You wish for sleep to get you once more and leave this world of hurt behind but it's not to be. When Barbara and I got up on that icy morning it was the silence, the terrible silence, which heralded and trumpeted our loss. It screamed *Craig is gone!! . . . He's not in his room! . . . He's dead and you'll never hear his voice again!*

Craig was the very life of our home and his not being there returned it to being merely a house. Everything that defined us had been stolen and what was left was a hollow, meaningless shell of existence. We walked into his room and looked at the toys and posters and all his beloved things. We looked at his bed—empty—and we said nothing. Pain, pain, pain, bloody pain. When we had our breakfast—a cup of tea maybe—we tried to talk over the silence but it wouldn't be ignored. That whole day, all I can remember is that silent, painful, empty nothingness that dripped from every wall and covered us. I think Barbara and I were at our worst that day. The fuss and bother—the circus—that had surrounded us and distracted us from the moment that Craig had died, was gone. We were left with our loss to cope with, with our life to live and it hit us so very hard.

Later that afternoon Barbara and I sat in front of the TV, not talking, not watching, just alone together in our thoughts. There was a knock at the door and in came my parents and my brother Darren. My mother had left her bag in the house and had come down to collect it. They came in and sat down but Barbara and I had nothing to give of ourselves. Barbara left and went up to the grave. Her own mother was up there in fact. I was left in the house but I just couldn't speak. I remember *Fletch* was on the TV and Darren trying to break the ice with a comment but I couldn't even respond. We all sat there and it was uncomfortable for them, I'm sure. I felt for them because I knew it was an incredibly awkward situation but there was nothing I could do—I was in my own inner world of excruciating pain.

They didn't stay long. They got up and said that they'd leave me be. I apologised, telling them I just wasn't able to talk. When they left I went up to Craig's room and cried my heart out. I was a broken man. I had nothing within to allow me to cope with this. There was nothing that was going to make this better, ever. It was relentless, hideous, all-consuming despair and there was nothing to be done about it.

Chapter 9 ∼
Moving On

It's fair to say that our lives were a mess after Craig had passed. We had no direction to follow and no will to live. We were so distraught and in such pain that getting out of bed was an immense achievement in itself. The silence in our house was our greatest enemy. As any parent knows, the noise and commotion of a youngster—playing with toys, watching TV, running in and out of the house—becomes an accepted background din in a home. It goes with the territory.

Craig often used to walk in circles around the sofa, playing with a car or plane in some imaginary setting, as we sat and watched TV. We never minded. We'd stopped noticing really, as you do. He'd often run a toy car along the back of the sofa, narrating some story as he went, and driving it over our heads and down our arms. We actually loved this; especially me. I found it very relaxing and therapeutic as the car was rummaged through my scalp. My eyes would begin to get heavy with mouth drooping open, complete with drool, as the massaging sensation of the wheels drew paths through my hair. Craig would sometimes get annoyed when I'd try to influence his narrative by suggesting the car remain on my scalp or shoulder 'to hide from enemy advances'. It would work once or twice only, before he'd cop to what I was at.

Barbara and I used to play another game with him too: we'd get him to brush our hair as we watched TV (of course the term *game* is used very loosely here!). I'd look over and watch Barbara's chin disappearing into her neck as Craig carefully brushed the long strands of hair. Then I'd interrupt, 'C'mon, it's my turn,' with Craig moving over then to brush mine. This would go back and forth for a while. Eventually our greediness got the better of us with my pleas of 'C'mon,

Craig, you did your mammy longer there. I need a couple more minutes' usually followed by Barbara's protests of 'No, he didn't!' while sneakily sniggering at me as Craig kept brushing. But Craig was always quick to put an end to this. 'Right, I'm not doing anyone's anymore now,' he'd say, and walk off. He was true to his word too— the only exception being a situation involving the exchange of money. Craig was a moralist . . . but a businessman too.

Those wonderful memories only drew tears now as we sat on our sofa in our empty, silent house. We found it hard to know what to do with our time, how to fill it. Time was our enemy. We wished it away but it was immovable. We both genuinely knew what it was to feel suicidal. We thought, individually and privately, how easy it would be to join Craig once more. If we chose to, we could be reunited with him in a matter of minutes. No impossibly long and barren future to mope through. This world held nothing for us now. It didn't. There was nothing in it that meant anything to us. I could see it in Barbara's eyes and she in mine. A few pills perhaps? It could be done so quickly. The very thought of it brought something close to excitement.

It's a terrible thing to want to end your life. It's a terrible dark state of mind to find oneself in, but here we were. There was only one thing that stopped us though, and it was Craig. Craig loved his life. He lived it, despite every setback, with the utmost joy. In spite of every difficulty, every illness, every unfavourable situation he found himself in, he'd push on through and keep smiling. It was his extraordinary ability to focus on the one positive in a rain of negatives that was so remarkable. How could Barbara or I take our own lives, when he struggled and battled for every second of his? In how he lived his short life he showed us how it was to be done. In how he lived his life, he saved ours.

But, with our decision made, we were left in this unwanted life. It was impossible to be motivated about anything. We were lost in every sense of that word. I remember thinking about my future soon after Craig had passed. The meaninglessness in everything was intolerable. Writing, music and creativity were my passion, nothing else. But when Craig died I lost everything. When he slipped from this world my only thought was, 'Where is he now?' Dreams and ambitions were all redundant and insensible to me. They abandoned my soul completely: those thoughts were just comprised of rubbishy, egotistical bullshit that was irrelevant. No, the philosophical mire I immediately found myself in was the only thing that existed. Finding out where my son was, what this life is all about, was my only concern.

Barbara had nothing, though. Whereas I became obsessed with any book I could get on the paranormal, life after death, after-death communication, fringe science and any esoteric philosophical schools of thought, Barbara looked nowhere. I was convinced that Craig had moved on to some other form of existence, but Barbara believed—or more accurately, feared greatly—that he was simply gone. For her there was no promise of seeing her boy again; just an empty void of non-existence. There was nothing in her life to pull her through. In our grief it was obvious that we were very different.

I simply couldn't have gone on if I was in any doubt that our beautiful, smiling and charismatic little Craig was still alive in some way. Once I believed this, once I knew this, I knew I had to do every-thing I could to find out where he'd gone. I just couldn't say to myself, 'Craig's dead. I need to grieve him and move on.' For me death was not finality. I knew, as I sat there crying at his grave, that he was alive somewhere. I just knew it. I had no proof. No evidence. But I knew. I loved my son too much to just leave it at that. I simply couldn't 'accept' he'd *probably* gone to some kind of heaven. I needed to know, needed to try and understand where or what that 'heaven' was. I'd never give up on him.

For me it was like what I can only imagine the parents of a kidnapped child feel. When their child is taken from them, they are compelled to search out his/her whereabouts. Despite all negative advice and overwhelming probabilities of that child's demise, the parents never give up. How can they when they simply do not know the truth? Those parents will often quote, 'It's the not knowing that's so hard.' That is how I felt and feel still. My son had gone to some new place and I knew nothing of it. I didn't know how he was coping or feeling 'there'. So here I was faced with the challenge of uncovering what I could of his whereabouts but not knowing where to begin. I genuinely didn't know what to do or indeed if there was anything I could do.

A couple of weeks after Craig's body had been buried Barbara and I decided to go to Edinburgh for a week. We just needed to get away from it all. Even that decision to go was laced with fear, guilt and pain. We didn't want to leave our little boy behind. The idea that we would not be at his grave for those days filled us with a terrible sense of guilt and hurt, even shame. We felt like we were already abandoning him. We fought with this until we finally decided that we needed to go. Getting up on the morning of our departure, we headed to the grave first and spoke with Craig. We told him where we were going and asked him to come along with us. We told him that he was free now to go where he wished and that we'd love to think he was there with us. We stayed for a while, then made our move.

In the airport itself the emptiness inside ate away at us. We remembered how Craig had been with us when we'd gone to Edinburgh just after Christmas the year before. The chill in the air and the seasonal festivities made this trip seem so similar, except for the glaring absence of our Craig. Every step of our journey to Edinburgh that day was laced with memories and pain.

When we got there it was terrible. We tried our best to clear our heads but it was impossible. The ghost of Craig was everywhere. I walked through the park and could see him walking by my side. I walked over to the playground and could see him on the bridge, in the hoop and on the swing. I walked into the old graveyard and saw Craig standing at the large tree where I'd photographed him in the cold and grey of that winter's day. I remembered the grey squirrel that we'd seen up in the tree. I remembered us meeting the man in the park who was feeding another squirrel. He had given Craig some food to try with the squirrel too. Everywhere I could see Craig and I cried with my head pressed down as I walked. I know people saw me—but what did I care? Shame was nothing when I'd lost everything.

Barbara walked around looking in the various shops but she saw nothing. Not like she used to. Rags on hangers and various tac was all that she could see now. The shallowness in all that was on display: the triviality of decoration and adornment. None of this meant a damn thing anymore.

When we met for our lunch on that first day we were two ghosts. I could see the emptiness behind Barbara's eyes. There was no rustling of bags or the quiet effervescence of enthusiasm and joy. No, it was a slow, heavy walk that approached to join me for lunch. We even questioned our being there.

We also uncovered a peculiar and horrifying new way of thinking while there. It had hit us both as we spent time alone walking around

Edinburgh that morning: we had nobody to worry about! We had no child to ring or text home to see if they were settling ok. We had no child to wonder how they were getting on while we were away. It was such a lonely and bleak new reality to accept. Our gorgeous little boy wouldn't be there to meet us at the airport or run up to us when we got home. His beautiful smile and bursting excitement would never *ever* be there to meet us. He was gone.

We had gone from being parents, from being a family, to being just a couple again like any other couple out there sitting in cafés and bars. The difference was they had hopes and dreams and the excitement of a life of opportunity. They sat and laughed and made plans. They laughed with the lightness of unburdened souls and melted happily into their surroundings. But we were just imposters in their world. We did not belong there. We no longer belonged anywhere, it seemed. We stood outside the window of life, in the rain, looking in at a world that kept moving. We were disjointed and displaced from normality and we hated it.

———

During that week in Edinburgh I knew I had to write a memorial piece for Craig. We wanted to have it in the paper before his Month's Mind Mass. But the prospect of putting pen to paper scared me, I have to say. Writing Craig's eulogy had been one of the most painful things I'd ever done so this was something I dreaded.

But eventually I headed to Starbucks and began the process. I sat there and all I could see was my beautiful little Craig. Memory after memory raced through my mind. My eyes welled with tears, my lips quivered and I forcefully stared out the window so that I could not be seen. My throat ached to roar but I suppressed it. I wrote some words and then hated what I was doing. I hated that it had come to this; that I was sitting there writing a pathetic tribute to my Craig when he should be just there with me. We'd been in that Starbucks together less than a year before. We'd sat and chatted about things that I couldn't remember: probably some idle nonsense that was meaninglessly wonderful for what it allowed—time with my son.

Every time I tried to write something I'd find myself getting caught up in a memory. I'd become distracted remembering his voice and visualising the expressions on his face. I'd hear his laughter and remember the warmth of his arm as he placed it round my neck. I'd remember how often he used to say 'I love you' to me and Barbara. All these emotions would flood my mind and not a single word was written. I just found it impossibly hard to do. I left.

But later that day I forced myself to face up to it, to live through it and get it done. I owed it to Craig. I sat for three hours crying and torturing myself until it was finished.

When we eventually saw that tribute in the paper our hearts were deeply pained. It was as if Craig's whole life and everything that he meant to us and those around him had been reduced to two pages in a local paper. It was so sad. Craig was not just another story to us. I think it was about this time that Barbara suggested to me that I write a book. I loved the idea but didn't think I could do it. I certainly couldn't do it at that time. I told Barbara that the pain was just too much to bear.

Our week in Edinburgh went slowly but ended too soon. There's no escaping the pain of grief and no matter where you are the loss is still the same. But that week in Edinburgh gave us some space to breathe and allowed us to be anonymous.

Leaving Edinburgh we had an uneasy feeling as we flew home. It was that uncomfortable truth that we were on our way home to that empty, silent house where misery and sadness awaited. The word 'home' didn't seem appropriate anymore either. Home is a place of comfort and sanctuary, an oasis of respite from the furious world. It is a place of love and loved ones. It is where families live as one and create and share memories together. What we were going back to used to be a home, but was not anymore. For us the true pain was knowing that this time our Craig wasn't waiting for us. He wouldn't be running towards us and leaping up into our arms with that unreserved and explosive display of love that children are so wonderful at. There would be no coy looks as he almost apologetically, but determinedly, asked 'What did ye get me?' Those eyes, those dimples, that wonderful smile and soft voice would not be there and never would be again.

When we got home we came in the door and met the silence head on. We said little as we rushed to turn on lights and the TV, desperately trying to bring noise and activity into the house. Sitting there in that house, back in Gorey, the weight of our loss seemed so much heavier. There was no distraction from our thoughts here, only their reinforcement. We were back in the mire, sinking with every breath. The memories, the loss, the pain all stared back out at us from every wall in every room. The TV sat in the corner of the living room yet our minds were drifting elsewhere; being pulled down dark and morbid alleys of persistent sorrow and inner turmoil. Our reality was a true nightmare.

Living in Gorey there was no escaping the oppression of our situation and everywhere we went there was a feeling that we'd become 'that couple who'd lost their child'. It was such a lonely, isolating feeling as we watched other people going about their business. We were the spectres among the living. Everywhere we looked life lived on. Shops were opening and people were commuting to work. Friends were gathering in coffee shops or bars and laughing at trivialities and nonsense. The hand on the clock ticked ever forward as people spoke on radio programmes, giving out about politicians or various injustices. How could they not know that our lives had come to an end? How could people just carry on with their frivolous, meaningless existence when the true nature of life eluded them, when at any minute they or their loved ones could face the horrors that we were enduring at that time? We felt so apart from the world. Life, living, was just some fragile, temporary mystery that duped us all. Its tune coaxed us along like some pied piper towards an inevitable end and we just danced and followed its lead. Unquestioning and unconcerned, we all moved in harmony to a deathly air.

As we walked around Gorey, or sat having tea in Joanne's coffee shop, there was always that feeling that people were perhaps looking over and pointing us out to their friends, saying 'God love them, that couple over there, see them, they just lost their son a few weeks ago.' Now, they probably weren't, to be honest, but it often felt that way. I remember not wanting to go up the town just in case I bumped into someone I knew. I really didn't want to face a sympathy talk or watch the discomfort of those who simply didn't know what to say.

They'd bump into us coming out of a shop or as we came round a corner and when they'd see our faces I could actually see the reality of the predicament they were in spread across their face. Neither we nor they wanted the encounter, but here we were. I always identified with those people. I was never one for those types of situations myself. I avoided them if I could. Every now and again we'd see someone up ahead of us in the distance and watch as they disappeared into a shop or side-street or just walk past looking the other way, pretending not to have seen us. Barbara was often hurt by this when she realised what had just happened. I always saw it differently, though. I was actually glad to have avoided the awkwardness. It suited me. But then I've always been a bit like that anyway. Barbara was always much more of a people person than me and she never shied away from meeting and talking with anyone. This is why it hurt her and not me. She was disappointed in those people for so obviously ignoring her. This made her feel like she was some kind of leper to be avoided. She really took it to heart and found it difficult to live with.

But we did have to live with it. In those early days the 'avoidance' was more prominent, but as time passed and people's perceptions of our state of grief changed, those who walked by now began to stop and speak with us. This actually eased the tension for us; for me especially. I was glad that we'd met most people and that the awkwardness of any future encounters was being dissolved. It cleared the air so to speak and paved the way for more natural and easy conversations when we'd meet these people again.

————

Craig's Month's Mind Mass was the next difficult affair. We had arrived early to the church and found ourselves a place in a pew near the front. We were sitting there just talking quietly to each other when Sister Breda, the Principal of Craig's school, came over to greet us. She extended her sympathies and then gave us a large parcel which she told us contained Craig's school books, copies and bits and pieces. We thanked her dearly and she left to find her seat. We were stunned by what was in our hands. Neither of us had even thought about retrieving his things from school so this was a real bolt out of the blue. How we hadn't even thought about it was a mystery to us both. But when I think back on those first few weeks, I can see that we were two lost souls with no coherence of thought or road to follow. We were completely at sea and all other thoughts that were not '*Craig is gone*' were obsolete and irrelevant to us. They simply weren't forthcoming at all.

Many months after that mass we discovered a little girl had been there. She was from Craig's school and apparently had held a torch for him. It was a lady from the school who told us in fact. She said that she had seen the little girl, with her parents, and she was dressed so pretty and looked so sad. We were both moved beyond measure when we heard this. We were also so very happy for Craig. We could almost picture him smiling and winking as he stood in the church watching the pretty little girl sitting there for him.

We never got to find out who that girl was but a couple of years later I'm pretty certain I got to see her. I had been standing at the foot of Craig's grave, but had my back to it as I spoke to another lady, Bernie, whose daughter Megan was buried opposite from Craig. We had been talking for a long time and although I had been aware of people walking past behind me on the footpath, I hadn't really paid any attention. I had just said goodbye to Bernie and turned around to kiss Craig goodbye when I noticed a small bunch of flowers laid neatly at the foot of the grave. They were wrapped in tinfoil and looked lovely. Immediately I knew they must have been left by some of the people who had gone past behind me. I looked around the graveyard as quick as I could and saw a lady and a young girl walking down the next row. The lady caught me staring at her and then quickly pointed to the girl at her side—it was she who had left the flowers. I don't know why, I think I was in a hurry to leave at that point, but I never went over to speak with them. I just called out 'thanks very much' and smiled at the girl. I should have gone over and thanked her personally and asked her name. I'm sure it was that little girl who had come to the church for Craig but I can never be certain.

——

Whilst writing this chapter I overheard a poet on the radio. I was coming back from the gym and was just about to change the station when I heard this guy mentioning bereavement. What he said resonated with me so profoundly that I want to mention it here. The presenter had quite casually asked him how he dealt with his bereavement, after losing his four-year-old child. The poet's reply was perfect. He corrected the presenter for applying the word 'bereavement' to any parent who loses a child. He said that 'bereavement' applies when we lose an elderly parent, a husband or wife, a sister or brother or perhaps a good friend. But bereavement doesn't apply when a parent loses a child. He said it was an 'apocalypse'. He was so right. Everything that applies to that word, applies to the loss a parent feels when their child dies. It is the end of all things. It is the end of time itself. Your reality changes in an instant and you are birthed into some new, foreign existence devoid of any meaning or point; but plentiful in pain, regret and sorrow. Your old life is no more and your new life is unwanted. So, after Craig died, and after all the ceremonies were over, we were still left to live our post-apocalyptic existence. Time moved on—and carried us reluctantly with it.

——

One day, just over a year after Craig had left us, I found myself out in the recently converted garage working on the new laptop I had. I was busy backing up a lot of family pictures and files from the old computer and was finding it very difficult as I sifted through old video clips and pictures of Craig. Hearing his voice was so wonderful and so painful at the same time.

As I finished backing up all those important treasures I sat back to think of what else could be lying around somewhere that needed to be saved. Leaning back and racking my brains I turned around to see the creative Zen player on top of a nearby shelf. Instantly, I remembered that I had recorded some stuff on the other Zen in the kitchen. I'd forgotten. I raced out to the kitchen and brought the Zen in to go through it. There was a series of recordings I had made while Craig was sick and while we were doing different things together. I backed them up immediately and then went through them.

I was a bit anxious about listening to them but I wanted to. As soon as I played the first clip I bawled. I heard Craig's voice speaking out at me but I was not prepared for what I heard. All the other clips I'd been watching and listening to were of Craig when his speech had been either normal or only moderately affected. But this recording was entirely different. Craig's voice came through the speakers and shook the bones in me. His speech was slurred and nasal and with every word he spoke I cried for the cruelty and injustice of it. Hearing just how bad his speech had been terrified and sickened me. I wanted to reach into the voice I was hearing and hug my Craig. I wanted to hold him and take it all back. I felt so guilty and useless as I listened to what had become of him.

The recording had been taken in my back room where Craig had been sitting on the office chair ordering particular Yu-Gi-Oh cards off eBay. He had just finished making his order and we were talking as we were about to leave the room. I had begun the recording while Craig was still sitting in his chair. The first words I heard when I listened back were those of Craig, who upon realising he was being recorded uttered, in his best DJ voice, the words 'Hi, you're through to 2FM—Join the line . . .' On the recording I was laughing at how quick Craig had been to come up with those improvised words, but sitting there in the room, listening, I was in tears. Craig then asked, 'What day is it?' to which I replied Wednesday, and to which he immediately remarked, 'Not long 'til Friday then, is it?' This was something that Craig used to say during the school week when he was looking forward to the weekend. It was a phrase that, to me, has since become synonymous with optimism, positivity and hope. It is forward thinking and focused, but will forever remind me of the first time I ever heard him saying it one night in bed, and how it had made me laugh so much. Craig had always made me and his mammy laugh with that sharp wit of his. It was a gift.

Sitting alone in the room I moved onto another recording. I was surprised at how long it appeared to be: it was fifty minutes in length. But that's when it hit me. Exactly ten days before Craig died I had made this recording as we went to bed one night. I knew then that this recording would be difficult to sit through. I paused for a moment, not because I was unsure of whether to listen to it or not—I knew I would —but to brace myself. I was already a blubbering mess and knew that this recording was going to be so very difficult to hear. I took a gulp and pressed Play.

I listened as Craig and I were slightly far off sounding. We were in the en suite, where I had Craig on my knee as I brushed his teeth, and we were chatting. The Zen was in the main room and that's why it sounded so far away. Then our voices came closer as I lifted Craig into bed and settled him on his pillow. This was prayer time and we began our nightly ritual straight away. The first thing I did was to place the green scapular around Craig's neck as we recited our prayers. Our Father, Hail Mary and then Craig did his own: 'St Brigid of Ireland help us we pray; for your love and your kindness we pray every day.'

Part of our nightly routine was Craig's feet, hands and face massage. He loved it. I listened on the recording as Craig sighed 'AAahhhh' while I rubbed the lotion over his feet and hands and he melted into the pillow. Then I went through some exercises with his hand and arm which were curled up to his shoulder because of the tumour. I stretched it out and Craig sighed 'Agghhhhh, that's lovely' as I continued to pull the arm right down to the fingers and stretch them out to the tips. We talked about his arm and I tried to explain why it was that way and how it would soon be back to normal once the signals from his brain were able to connect to it again. I tried to explain that the wires (his nerves) going from his head to his arm were being blocked by the lump and that as soon as the lump went it would be fine again. I also showed him some exercises that he could do with his fingers that could help to teach his brain to reconnect everything again. I got him to touch his thumb off each of the fingers of that hand over and over again, back and forth, and said that if he remembered to try that a few times each day, it would help.

When we were finished with that I washed my hands and moved to his face, where I used to pretend to paint it. Craig loved this. This was something I used to do if he was hyper or couldn't sleep. I used to pretend my left hand was an easel and then I'd dip my right hand index finger into its palm and move it back to paint across his face. I'd narrate, in a very low, grumbly voice:

'Okay . . . just get a little bit of blue here . . .' (then I'd rub my finger across his eyebrows) '. . . now a little touch of red . . .' (as I quickly dipped the finger back in the easel and returned to stroke down across the forehead and down by the temples. I'd watch as Craig's face would become heavy and still, completely relaxed by the low voice and sweeping movements across his face) '. . . Now maybe a little bit of indigo to accentuate the lower eye . . .' (dipping into the hand again and then gently applying the colour to the lower ocular area.) I'd repeat this routine across his face and eyelids until he was completely still and almost on the verge of sleep. This would usually be enough and I'd slip off out of the room to leave him sleep; job done. But occasionally

I'd go to make my exit only to see Craig's little pursed lips barely move in saying 'I'm not asleep yet . . . just a little bit more?'—every other muscle in his face and body perfectly still. In those instances I'd go through a 'wiping' routine where I'd remove the paint with slow, deliberate thumb strokes, ' . . . and now I just need to wipe away this bit, and this little bit . . . and maybe a little bit over here . . . and another little bit just under here . . .' (I'd wet the pad of my thumb for some 'stubborn' areas—usually the eyelids—just to add another refreshing element to the mix.)

On the recording Craig enjoyed this for a while but was still awake afterwards so I had climbed into the bed and we talked. We played another favourite game of ours which was 'guess the song'. Here we would take turns in humming a tiny part of a song, with the other having to guess what it is. This was usually when the giggles kicked in as tunes were deliberately hummed in the most inadequate and grotesque manner so as to make guessing impossible—and to of course incite the hysteria. Listening to the recording it was such a joy to hear Craig in fits of giggles as he hummed a tune that I had no idea of. He was so far gone that he couldn't even hum the tune without cracking up completely. As I listened I remembered it well.

We played that game for a while but then I seemingly grabbed the remote controls and began to sift through the different channels on the TV for him to watch. As I listened I remembered how Craig had taken the Zen mp3 in his hand at the time. On the recording there was a silence. In that silence Craig was looking at the picture of himself that was on the front screen of the Zen. He was looking at it and he was thinking. The silence lasted for about ten seconds until it was broken by Craig making some very low, mumbling noises—he was talking to himself, with the mp3 microphone very close to his mouth. Then I began speaking about what was on the TV, clearly not having heard what Craig was after saying to himself.

Before listening to anymore I decided to rewind the recording to see could I make out what, if anything, Craig had been mumbling. I turned the volume right up and put my ear to the speaker. The beginning and end of his words I could not make out but the bit in the middle, when I listened, broke my heart. I erupted in tears as the words pierced me: 'I can't wait to talk to my friends, to laugh and to run again.'

The words haunted me as I listened to the pain they hid. They rang out crystal clear and I hated myself for not hearing them the first time while he was lying next to me. He had spoken from his heart and I never heard. Craig had always kept his pain from us. He never really ever spoke about his worries, only on rare occasions. Those words revealed so much.

After listening to those heartfelt words from Craig I stopped the recording and cried for about ten minutes. I wanted to hold him in my arms and love him. I wanted to say sorry for not protecting him, for not keeping him safe. I was so angry that he was taken from us and in the way he was taken. When I finally composed myself I continued to play the recording.

But within only a matter of seconds I was gone again. Craig's voice, out of nowhere and out of any context, turned to me and said, 'Daddy . . . Ye know I love you, don't you?' I immediately collapsed into my hands and cried my eyes out. I cried loudly, uncontrollably, as those words rang in my ear and I thanked the heavens that I had made that recording. It was so beautiful to hear them coming from his voice. It was the most glorious sound in the world. My response on the recording was nowhere near as profound as the reaction I was having while listening. The pain of Craig's parting was not yet in the voice of the man I heard. I merely replied 'I know it with all my heart, darling,' and never even told him that I loved him back. *God, why didn't I just say that.*

Craig then paused on the recording. 'I'm so well there, amn't I?' he said quietly.

'You're looking at the picture there, are you?' I replied on the recording, as I remembered leaning into him and looking at the screensaver image of Craig's beautiful, smiling face looking back at us. It had been taken the previous Christmas when we were in Edinburgh, when Craig had been running around the park, healthy and full of energy. 'Well, keep looking at it 'cos that's the way you'll be again.'

'My two eyes were working,' he said, his voice breaking and the tears now filling up. 'I'm so ugly.'

'No, you're not!' I said, as I pulled myself to him.

'Yes I am!' he cried, 'I'm ugly.'

As I listened to this recording the tears were streaming down my face. It was so difficult to listen to him suffering such emotional torment. Memories flooded back of the times Barbara and I would catch Craig looking at himself in the mirror. We'd see him making faces and watch as only one side moved. He'd be so upset but seldom made a big to-do about it. But we knew. Craig's spirit, in those moments, was buckling and he'd become quiet. Sometimes we'd catch him looking out the window too at the other kids on the estate playing outside while he held some toy or cards in his hands, all by himself. Those were the moments where he felt so alone, so different, so excluded.

'Look at me, Craig,' the recording continued, as I sought to ease Craig's worries. 'You will look like that again, do you hear; just as soon as that lump is gone, ok!'

'No, I won't. I'm always going to be ugly! I'm just an ugly fucker.' Craig was so upset.

'You're *not* ugly!' I repeated. 'You're beautiful and always will be beautiful, do you hear me. I wish I looked like you. Look at me . . . I'm a big ugly FUCKER, the big head on me.'

Craig began to laugh a little as soon as I said that. I remember being relieved at the time. I listened to Craig's chuckles and I felt a smile on my lips.

'No you're not,' Craig said. 'I think you're a big nice chappy.'

'Well, I think you're a lovely chappy, Craig,' I replied, before quickly adding 'Do you know what Craig, I think we're both lovely chappies.'

'Well, I think *you're* a lovely chappy.' He meant it. He said it twice because he wanted me to know it. Here Craig was being so typically him. It was he who had the demons to deal with and yet here he was reaching out to me, trying to make me feel better.

I could feel the power of his spirit on that recording; the depths of it. I was filled with so much admiration and respect for the boy who was part of me, part of Barbara, but who was and is so much more. That recording captured his tears, his laughter and his unquestionable strength. One of the last things on the recording was how I half-heartedly spoke to Craig about the strong language he was using. Barbara and I had kind of turned a blind eye to any swearing Craig had been doing in the previous few weeks. In truth, I probably encouraged it and, more often than not, instigated it. It made Craig laugh and that was always going to be so much more important to us than anything else. On the recording I listened as Craig jokingly swore here and there, his preferred word always being *fucker*, and how I took him to task on it:

'Listen, what are we going to do about all this bad language, eh?' I asked, after Craig had used the *fucker* word more than normal.

Silence from Craig. Immediately I must have regretted bringing up the subject because the silence was only finally broken by me as I said 'Although it's a great word isn't it—*fucker!*'

Straight away Craig began to giggle. 'Yeah,' he said. '*Fucker*—it goes so smoothly, doesn't it?' as he giggled yet again at the power of its sound.

I laughed as I listened to him.

_____

I must have played the above sections of the recording at least twenty times that evening; the words piercing so deeply within me. It was painful but addictive—and there were of course all those treasured words too. But in the time since that night, I've played that recording only once or twice. There is joy in it, and there is pain. For the moment the pain is too great though. It hurts me to listen to Craig in such an advanced state of his illness. It hurts me to remember; to relive. But within the anguish there is so much love to be heard and felt. Barbara still hasn't been able to listen to the recording. It's just too much for her and I don't blame her. I had to listen to it when writing this part of the book and all I could do was cry—again.

But I'm glad that I've listened to it. It is one of my most prized possessions. It has reminded me, shown me, how wonderful my son is. You see, through the pain, through the tears, through the oppressive torment Craig's light shines through. Most of that recording is laughter—Craig's laughter. Through the disfigurement, the disablement, the inner fear and tears of pain he suffered, Craig still laughed and giggled and never allowed his spirit to be crushed. He was not safeguarded from those darker thoughts—he felt them and buckled under them. But he always pushed back. That was his strength. That is why we are so incredibly proud of our son. I'll never forget those words, though it pains me that I never heard them the first time. Words that were quietly said to himself; words that showed his pain but ultimately his resolve and true spirit: 'I can't wait to talk to my friends, to laugh and to run again.'

_____

One of Craig's most endearing qualities was his ability to reach out to others. His empathy and emotional intelligence was extraordinary and so he could always feel out a situation and adapt. He was also guided by an inherent sense of what was right and wrong and often stepped in to help others who needed it. I can think of one example of this straight away . . .

Reaching Out

Craig came home from school one day and told us about something that happened during the morning and which troubled him. He was annoyed at what some boys had done and wanted to get our opinion on it, so he explained to us what had happened. He had been on his lunch break, playing outside in the yard with his friends, when he noticed a smaller boy being hassled by some bigger ones. 'He's only a new boy,' Craig told us, as he conveyed the concern that led to his ultimate reaction, 'and it wasn't fair that those bigger boys were annoying him,' he continued.

We didn't know where this was leading but then Craig told us. 'I just walked over and told them other boys to leave him alone, and told the new boy that he could play with me,' he said. Barbara and I were so proud. 'It's not nice when you don't know anybody and those other boys were just being horrible.'

It was such a brave thing to do really. Craig was a big chap, but that doesn't always mean much in the school playground. I know Craig was thought of highly among his friends and so he had a good bunch to rely on too. But still, it takes guts to step in like he did and it really is a measure of the man he was and is still.

Another example of Craig's friendly nature came to our attention only after he died. Just a few days after Craig passed away we received a beautiful card in the letterbox. It was from a neighbour Mary-Claire, whom we didn't even know of at the time. She sympathised with our loss but then went on to tell us a little story about our Craig. She wanted to get across just how grateful she was for something that he had done; something we knew nothing of. You see she had a son, Harry, who was over two years younger than Craig, and who lived around the corner from where most of the other kids used to hang out. She explained the reason why she was so thankful to Craig: he was the first child to ever call to her door and ask to play with her son. She had been so chuffed at the time, and loved him for it.

When Barbara and I read that card we were moved to tears. It was exactly like Craig to do something like that. He was such a people person and treated everyone the same. It turned out that Mary-Claire and I actually knew each other, having gone to the same primary school in Bray together. Her son Harry, and Craig, ended up attending the same Montessori in Gorey too—Higgy's House—and so they got to know each other pretty well.

After Craig passed away Higgy's House were kind enough to plant a beautiful copper beach tree at the front of their premises in tribute to Craig. It was a beautiful gesture which Barbara and I are forever thankful for, and on the day they organised a small ceremony to mark the occasion. Words and poems were read out while we stood around the tree and remembered Craig together. Mary-Claire was there too and she told us yet another wonderful tale about our Craig. She laughed as she remembered how Craig used to occasionally call to the house asking for Harry to come out, but that sometimes Harry would be in the middle of his dinner. Mary-Claire would tell Craig this and let him know that Harry would only be out afterwards. But then, while she and the family continued to sit and have their dinner together, they'd hear a voice talking intermittently through the letterbox—'Harry! . . . Are you finished your dinner yet?' . . . . Patience was perhaps not Craig's greatest attribute!

Another parent, very recently in fact, also shared something very touching with us about Craig. Her son and Craig were in the same class and they were good friends. Craig had even been to this boy's house for a birthday party and they enjoyed each other's company a lot. But what we didn't know, and were only told years after Craig's passing by this boy's mother, was that her son prior to meeting Craig was quite withdrawn and introspective, to the point where they were actually concerned about him. However, as soon as this boy met Craig he began to transform.

She told us how relieved they were as they watched him slowly come out of himself and open up more. All she remembers hearing was Craig's name and then, when she met him at her son's birthday party, she was completely enamoured by him.

I actually remember, very well, the evening that I called around to collect Craig from that party. I arrived at the same time as some other parents and we all stood in the hallway waiting for our kids to appear. I can remember standing there with the other mums and dads and then being approached by the boy's mother. She had made a point of coming straight to me and telling me how wonderful Craig had been. 'He was the life and soul of the party,' she said. I was chuffed and so very proud. 'He's just so funny and he had everyone in stitches,' she continued. I felt privileged to be singled out like this. I hadn't known anybody there and was made to feel so very comfortable and extremely proud of my son.

But knowing that Craig had helped others in the way that he did—by being strong and caring; by being himself—fills our hearts with fervent pride and we love him all the more.

Chapter 10

The Boy Who Lives

Not long after we came back from Edinburgh our thoughts turned to Christmas, which was only a matter of weeks away. In Edinburgh, as well as back home in Gorey, the festive season was in full swing. But with Craig gone we wanted no part in it.

When Craig first came into our lives the real magic of Christmas had come alive once more. For me it was the wonderment shining in his eyes that fuelled something long embered within. It burned fiercely in Craig. I cannot begin to recall the number of times I've read *The Night before Christmas* to Craig . . . and not just at Christmas either. We'd lie together in his bed with Craig snuggling into me as we went through each verse and flicked through the wonderfully evocative images.

Barbara remembers how excited Craig used to be when it came to putting the decorations up each year. He'd become giddy and dance on the spot as he helped with the various boxes that came down from the attic. 'Oh, Mammy,' he'd say, 'I love this. It's Christmas, it's Christmas, it's Christmas!' He'd bubble over, clasping his hands together and moving fitfully up and down on his heels. He'd help unload the boxes and look at all the ornaments as they were carefully removed. When the Christmas tree went up he'd even help with putting the decorations on. Although Barbara equally remembers how it wasn't long before he'd say 'This is boring, I'll leave you to do it,' and then walk away to do something—anything—more interesting.

And then of course there were his letters to Santa, penned at the dining room table. He'd be on my knee, excitedly shaking one of his crossed feet as he stared into the air thinking of what he wanted from Santa.

Little moments like these are what Christmas is all about.

———

Generally speaking everyone knows that Christmas really is a time for kids, but when you have a child of your own it really does reawaken that inner child. It allows you to feel the true wonder of Christmas once again. So facing our first Christmas without Craig was a terrifying prospect. We wanted to sleep and wake up to find that the whole period had been and gone. There is no time of year that is more family focused than Christmas. It is the one time of year where people scrabble for last minute flights home or fight for time off work just so as they can be with their loved ones. For Barbara and me our family had been ripped apart. There were no celebrations to be had; Christmas didn't exist for us anymore.

Losing a child is incomparable to anything else. In a lifetime where emotions and feelings are learned through such varied and diverse experiences, there is simply nothing that can prepare you for the total annihilation of your being that happens when your child dies.

So, with Christmas fast approaching we needed to make a decision. All we knew is that we didn't want to spend it in Gorey—but it wasn't as easy as that either. I was adamant that I needed to be around so that I could visit Craig's grave on Christmas morning. I couldn't contemplate not being there on that morning, of all mornings. Barbara didn't feel as strongly about that though. She really just wanted to run away from Christmas altogether and I could understand that too. Strange, considering it was always I who used to console Barbara with, 'He's not in that grave, he's somewhere free and happy'; there was something about Christmas Day that I just couldn't allow to come and go without us being at his graveside. Our task therefore was to find somewhere which wasn't too far away from Gorey so we could visit the grave, but where we could also spend the Christmas period alone and away from all the trappings of that time. After many searches I finally found a place—a log cabin in the Wicklow Mountains. But before we got there we still had to run the gauntlet of the pre-Christmas madness.

We couldn't go anywhere without being swamped by the endless songs and jingles that go hand in hand with the time of year. We spent a lot of our time just going for drives and heading up to different shopping centres. We just needed to get out of the house but we were limited to the places we could go to. There are only so many drives you can go on before they become tedious and there are only so many times that you can visit the same places before they start to do your head in. But as tedious and head-wrecking as these all were, they were a thousand times better than staying within the four walls of our house. There was just no way that we could spend our days sitting in, watching that bloody TV and getting under each other's feet. Time moved too slowly there. So, Christmas or not, we simply had to get out.

But it was painful. We both felt it: children running around with their parents, pointing out all the different toys that they wanted; the cheerful, merry Christmas music that played everywhere like some sick soundtrack to the horror that was our lives. We'd sit and have our lunch or just walk around the shops and watch as the gift-buying masses spilled in and out of every shop entrance clutching bags of folderol and whatnot, excitedly chattering and planning and blissfully lost in the atmosphere of Christmas cheer. But it was always the young families—who seemed to appear everywhere—that pained us most to see. They *were* us. They were what we *used* to be and what we should *still* be. We'd see a little boy, about Craig's age, and watch as he darted energetically around his parents. We'd only glance—but it was enough. The tremendous feeling of sadness and loss was a constant battle for us.

This was a side of Christmas I'd never seen or understood before. Growing up you'd often hear certain people talking about how they hated Christmas and how it was such a lonely time. I never could understand that: for me it was always magic and warmth. But now I realised that it was only ever those things to me because of the people who made it that way. It was being in the company of those whom you love that made Christmas so special. With Craig gone, Christmas had become the saddest time of all. Now I felt the loneliness that others spoke of: God, how I felt it. It paralysed me. Barbara, of course, had known sadness at Christmas before. The loss of her brother and father had always made it feel emptier. But none of that loss, none of those feelings could have ever prepared her for what hell she had now to live through.

———

Before we finally got to escape to the cabin, something quite extraordinary happened. It happened on 22 December in fact, but the story really begins on the day before this. On this particular day I was on my own in the house, with Barbara having gone to the hairdresser's. This was the first time that Barbara and I had actually been apart from each other since Craig died, so being on my own in the house I felt a certain amount of freedom to let go of my emotions. After she left I walked around the house looking at all the pictures of Craig and spending time in his room. I was very emotional, remembering all the wonderful times we had together and thinking of the future that was denied us—denied Craig. But it wasn't until I stood in the kitchen that I really let go.

My mind was filled with confusion as to where my little boy was and I became consumed with worry and fear. I literally broke down in tears, crying out to Craig to let me know that he was ok, somehow. As I cried out to Craig I was facing the ceiling. I begged him to find some way of sending us a message to help us cope with his 'death'. As I looked up at the light fixture overhead, containing four separate bulbs, I had a thought. 'Oh, darling, if you could even just blow that bulb,' I pleaded, as I pointed to one specific bulb out of the four that were there. I was inconsolable and needed something desperately to hold on to. I walked over to the light switch and turned the kitchen light on. I stood there waiting, but nothing happened. All the bulbs remained lit. I leaned against the kitchen sink just staring at those lights but nothing happened. I was so dejected, but at the same time, almost laughed at myself for thinking that it would. I dried my tears and walked away.

The very next day, however, after being out shopping for groceries, Barbara and I came into the kitchen with our bags. We threw the bags on the counter top and were just talking away to each other. It was quite a darkish day so Barbara turned and asked me to flick the lights on. When I did, the extraordinary happened. In the instant of my pushing that switch a loud explosion occurred and Barbara screamed as we both involuntarily covered our heads with our hands. The kitchen floor and counter top were completely covered in shards of broken glass as we cowered in complete shock. That's when it hit me. I looked up at the light and could barely believe my eyes when I could see that the bulb I had pointed out the previous day was no longer there. Not any other bulb, just the specific one that I had begged Craig to blow. It had completely exploded, like nothing I've ever witnessed or seen in my life, and all that was left was the metal base which was stuck in the light fixture. I had a surge of excitement running through me then. I flustered my words as I rushed to tell Barbara what happened the previous day and thus the significance of what had just happened that very second. I ran into the sitting room and grabbed Craig's picture from the mantelpiece and kissed him. I looked at the picture and gave Craig the thumbs up for literally 'blowing up' the bulb. I thanked him so much and told him that he was the most extraordinary person I'd ever known and that I loved him so much.

Barbara and I laughed as we pictured Craig saying, 'Right, well, if you want me to blow it . . . I'll bloody *blow* it all right!' He had left no room for doubt.

That was, I believe, the first communication that Barbara and I received from Craig since his departure from this world. But it was only to be the first of many extraordinary messages from Craig. Messages that came from the afterlife and that cemented for me, and for Barbara, our belief that our beautiful boy Craig is alive and well in some strange non-physical world that science cannot, yet, explain. The next communication we were to receive from Craig came very soon—within a couple of days of the 'exploding bulb' in fact. It was a different, entirely subjective form of communication, but a communication nonetheless.

––––

On 23 December, the time finally came for us to go to the log cabin. The view from its main window was breathtaking and we just hadn't expected it. It looked out over green fields and forestry and the beautiful Glenmalure Valley. In truth we would have been happy with a hut: as long as it was warm, dry and kept us away from Christmas.

Looking around, our first thoughts were the same, *Craig would've loved it here.* And he would. He would have been so excited: the location, the views, the unusual cabin and staying up late watching movies would have him in a spin. But our stomachs churned with the very thought of it: *Here we were having a new experience in a beautiful place* that Craig will never know about or who'll never be part of our memories here. It was the thought that we were building those new memories—without him—that hurt so badly.

Christmas Eve proved to be a very difficult and teary affair for us both. We sat in front of the TV that night trying our best to drown out the thoughts of what we should be doing were Craig with us still. The memories played in our heads of all the Christmas Eves before and how animated and fired-up Craig had always been. Our minds filled with images of his smiling face and the warmth of his little arms as he hugged us both. How he'd put out a single mince pie and a glass of milk for Santa and leave a couple of carrots for Rudolf and the other reindeers (originally I used to put out just one carrot, only to hear Craig's protest of, 'What about the other reindeers . . . they'll be hungry too!') In bed we'd read *The Night before Christmas* and then whisper excitedly together about Santa and all things Christmassy. There was enchantment in the air and we all felt it.

But sitting in the cabin that night, there was no magic; only that cold emptiness that had hijacked our lives. We sat for as long as we could but eventually couldn't take it anymore. We headed to our bed, looking for the darkness to take us away from the pain of our waking lives and away from the thoughts that betrayed us.

We both slept uneasily that night before waking very early and making our way down to Craig's grave. We wanted to get there as quickly and as early as we could. When we arrived there were only a couple of other people in the graveyard. It was cold and it was miserable. We crouched either side of his mucky grave and told him over and over again just how much we loved him and that we were so sorry for allowing this to happen to him. We placed a beautiful ornamental figure, that we'd bought in the 'Christmas Shop' in Edinburgh, on his grave and told him it was our little Christmas present to him.

There's an awareness that comes over you sometimes when you find yourself in certain situations, as if you are standing outside yourself watching your life as an observer might. While we knelt there, largely alone in a graveyard, placing a Christmas present on top of our son's grave that awareness came to us both: it was Christmas morning and here we were—two utterly destroyed people—in some bleak graveyard looking down at a mound of earth which concealed the body of our beautiful dead son. In that moment the enormous feeling of despair, the realisation of the absolute tragedy of our lives, tore at us. I lost any ability to speak as my throat, all swollen with suppressed, boiling emotions, seized up and my eyes welled up their tears. My chin shuddered uncontrollably as I watched and listened to Barbara spilling her tears freely, crying out for her little boy. It was a nightmare: an absolute nightmare.

We stayed for as long as we could but when it came time to leave we found it very difficult. It was everything against our hearts to walk away from our son on that day. But it isn't our son, I'd say to Barbara—to myself too. He's not there, he's alive someplace else. This was all that I could say. I didn't know that of course. It's just what I believed. It's what I had to believe if any of this was to make sense at all. The pain of walking away came with us and we drove back to the mountains with little to say to each other. We were lost in thought; lost in anguish.

We had a long day ahead of us on that day but at least, in the cabin, it didn't feel like Christmas that much. The new surroundings and the remote location lent itself to a feeling of being away and it provided a shelter from the torment of excited children noisily running outside with their new toys. In the cabin we were cocooned from all that. We spent the day watching films and specials on the TV and eating and drinking. We tried to distract ourselves as much as possible. When it came to eating Christmas dinner (which I'd collected from my mother) we filled a plate for Craig and set it at the table with us. We still do that now in fact. We'll never stop doing that, because we know he is with us, always.

It was after that dinner that 'something' happened which was extra-ordinary. I remember I was feeling particularly tired and uncomfortable and so I decided to go into our bedroom for a lie down. When I lay down I just started to cry. I was overwhelmed with such indescribable sorrow that I felt weak and powerless and the tears just flowed. As I lay there I eventually began to feel very sleepy and noticed how my limbs and extremities became comfortably heavy and warm. I was in that half-awake half-asleep state and I just lay there, still. It was just then that I had the most incredible experience. It was a dream but not exactly a dream either because I knew I was half-awake but nonetheless Craig appeared in front of me smiling and simply staring at me. He then slid his hand over the back of mine and continued smiling that wonderful peaceful smile at me. I could see his beautiful dimples and his gorgeous blue eyes. It was crystal clear and real. He never said a single word the whole time but I was overcome with a warm feeling of closeness. It was such a beautiful feeling to see Craig and feel his hand on mine. But just as I began to really soak it all in, the room became more dominant in my periphery and Craig began to slip away. I 'woke' then, although this is not the right word, and all I could think of saying was 'Thanks, Craig'. It felt so different to a dream and I took it that way. To me, I didn't know how (I didn't know anything anymore), but it *was* Craig who had come to visit to show me he was alive and well.

I lay there for another while hoping desperately that I could get back in touch with him. But the more I wanted it, the more awake I became until finally I had to give up. I went straight outside and told Barbara about it. I questioned out loud whether it actually had been Craig and we talked about it, briefly. Neither of us wanted to rationalise it and take away its power by talking and convincing ourselves that it 'had' to be a dream. But I knew, because I'd experienced it, that it wasn't.

———

The implication of this communication, and that involving the exploding bulb, for my understanding of the known world was astonishing. There were two thoughts that ran through my mind. The first was that I one hundred percent believed that my son had shown me evidence of some other 'realm', and which therefore meant I simply had to do everything in my power to try and understand and reach out to this place. Unlike the initial and continuing heartfelt *belief* I held in some continuation after death, these communications represented a compelling subjective proof that fired up my left logical brain into a frenzy of possibilities. I couldn't just turn away from this staggering truth and pretend life was as it seems. The second, and the most crucial of all, was the inference that came with my son's communication: Craig was ALIVE. He was residing in a hidden world where he was still capable of (albeit in a limited fashion) interacting with this one. Craig had shown us that he could bridge these worlds and communicate to us so it seemed to me that there had to be some chance that I could try and reach him too. There was some common ground where we could meet and this was something I was going to spend my life trying to do.

Those first communications opened up my mind to the intoxicating hope that I may, in my lifetime, find some way of reaching Craig. The feeling that I may have within some element of my control even a remote chance of finding him offered an incredibly powerful and rousing motivation for my own personal quest into understanding the real truth of life—and of infinitely greater importance . . . finding Craig. This was, is and always will be a path that I'm committed to walk.

I have read so many books since Craig passed on all manner of concepts pertaining to life after death with various coherent and contrasting theories as to the fundamental nature of what we call consciousness. Consciousness is after all the great mystery: Are we merely the sum of our parts? Does consciousness burn bright simply because of the many billions of neurons that fire countless signals within an evolutionarily formed complex brain? Or does consciousness survive death—the resulting implication being we are far more than the biology that resides in the physical?

I have read many books which seek to incorporate the mysterious shortfalls and bizarre implications of Quantum Physics into various subjective theories as to the possible nature of the universe, and how we as humans fit in with it all. In as much as science largely dismisses or ignores anything that falls outside what is conventionally acceptable within its own demarcation, and thus distances itself from all things alternative and paranormal, I am always drawn to those seekers of complete knowledge who embrace the rigours of a *true* scientific approach. Science was never about being an 'establishment' but an intellectual pursuit of knowledge and understanding. It may well be flawed by a combination of its peer approved structure and its competitive grant system but it's the elegance in its fundamentally experimental approach to understanding nature that has brought humanity so far in such a short time. Observation and experimentation have been the cornerstone of science, the discipline through which intellectual and technological advancement have been achieved. Those inspirational ideas and thoughts from the minds of our greatest scientists have been allowed to crystallise into our accepted reality through these disciplines. This is why I've always aligned myself with the purity of this methodology.

Like most I have always mistrusted, distanced myself from and shook my head at anything that is built upon nothing more than blind, unchallenged belief. Anything that requires me to put my head in the sand and ask no questions is abhorrent to me. It is not my way, nor ever will be.

But I have found myself in the most desperate and claustrophobic dilemma. I am looking to science to help me find my son but conventional established science really doesn't want to know. There are only a tiny inappreciable minority of respectable and able scientists looking into this so called 'fringe science' and who, by bravely doing so, inherently risk the condemnation and patronising slurs of their 'peers'. It is clearly the fear of this chastisement and of a 'career destroyed' that deters so many great scientists from giving the might of their intellect to this field. And it is we who are all the poorer for it. Certainly every parent out there who's ever lost a child is. You see I am certain after reading so much anecdotal evidence, and more crucially from my own direct experience of Craig communicating with us, his parents, that he is alive and well but in a way that I just do not understand yet. However, understanding this reality is really only secondary to the 'knowing' that Craig has already blessed us with. We know thanks to Craig's amazing connection that he lives on. His amazing soul has overcome the improbable odds that have turned aside so many others and has reached out to bring peace and comfort to his mammy and daddy.

I wanted to give examples in the next few pages of some of those messages that have shown us that there is life after death; that our Craig and the children of so many other grieving parents out there are alive and well and it is, therefore, only an interim before we will meet our children again. Some of the following examples will resonate more strongly, while others will appear dubious. That cannot be helped. The logical mind will always seek to find the most rational, most likely, explanation in all situations. There's a principle known as *Occam's Razor* which in basic terms states that the most simplistic hypothesis for explaining an unknown should be adopted ahead of an equally plausible but more complex one. I couldn't agree more. It is the quickest and most effective way of reaching a true understanding of anything. You will read the examples that follow and will apply your own *Occam's Razor* and rightly so. In every single case you will probably entertain more plausible reasons for what happened than what we would have you believe. But there is nothing I can do to affect that. That it is not my objective in putting these examples here. I do so because they are what happened to us. They are an account of various communications which WE are certain are from our beautiful Craig and in sharing them may, and should, help other grieving parents out there who are looking for some answers. I hope they help.

Happy Birthday, Mammy. . .

After the amazing incident of the 'exploding bulb' and my dreamlike visit from Craig the next communication we received from him came on Tuesday, 9 January 2007. It was Barbara's birthday and, despite not wanting to celebrate it, we decided to go out for a meal in Dublin. We booked a table in a city-centre restaurant and arrived in the evening for our meal. After placing our orders we sat back and waited for our starters to come. We were chatting away about something or other when I suddenly felt a really cold sensation around me. I didn't say anything, until Barbara shrugged her shoulders and said, 'Jesus where did that cold come from?' I, very sardonically, raised my knife in a mock levitation and made a 'spooky' noise, implying that we were being haunted. At that very moment, with the knife still in mid-air, *She will be loved*—a song that Craig loved so much—played over the speakers. I stopped in my tracks. We both looked at each other. We sat there numb. We were misty eyed as we sat and listened and thought of Craig singing the words, as he so often did.

'He's saying Happy Birthday to you,' I said to Barbara. It was a powerful moment. When the song was over, the first thing we both noticed was that the room became warm again. It was this, almost more than the music alone, that really convinced us that our Craig had come to say Happy Birthday to his mammy. We were so happy and yet so upset too. But it was another incredible feeling, knowing that Craig had just been communicating with us again.

Are You There Sidney? . . .

Only a week or so after Barbara's birthday, we received another signal from Craig. It was mid January and Barbara and I were feeling especially low. January is always a tough time and can be depressing, but when you've just lost your child it brings with it an excruciating bleakness that stifles you with a morbid defeatism. Add to this the fact we were beginning a new year with unemployment and were therefore lost in every way possible, we were pretty much the lowest we'd been since Craig had died. There was such sadness and incredible tension between us on this particular day. We were biting each other's heads off all evening in fact until eventually we were too weak to even do that.

We both sat on the couch in the sitting room and finally began talking about our despair. Barbara was inconsolable as she revealed how she just couldn't cope without Craig. She began crying hysterically and I held her as my own tears came rushing down my face. We were destroyed. It was at this precise moment, at the peak of our outpour, that the lamp in the corner of the room began to flicker on and off. It was the very same as you would see in a horror film. We stopped breathing. We just stared at the lamp and watched as it continued to flicker and dim back and forth, casting shadows on the walls. 'Is that you, darling, are you here?' we cried out. It flickered for another minute or so and we just watched and absorbed the significance. We spoke out to Craig, telling him we loved him and then it just returned to normal. We were so elevated by that encounter. It immediately brought us a sense of connection to Craig and a feeling of undying hope. It was a transformational experience in every conceivable way and we basked in it for a long time after.

I'm Behind You . . .

On 31 January we had our next visit from Craig. Barbara and I were in the house after spending the whole day sanding doors and doorframes. It was early evening time and I was vacuuming all the downstairs rooms to remove the dust and mess that was everywhere. Barbara had gone upstairs and had jumped into the shower.

I had moved from the kitchen out into the hall and was vacuuming up near the front door with my back facing the bottom of the stairs. I was vigorously trying to vacuum some of the more stubborn dust that was imbedded in the front door mat when Barbara came behind me and tugged at the back of my sweater. I turned around to see what she wanted, but she wasn't there. There was nobody there. I just stood there in disbelief, with the vacuum still running. I kept staring at the stairs. I looked to see was there anything or anyway that something could have caught the back of my sweater but there wasn't. I mean there *really* wasn't. I'm the worst person in the world for dismissing this type of thing and latching on to the most likely cause, but in this instance there was *nothing* that could account for that very obvious, human, tug on my shirt.

It hit me hard then. With tears in my eyes, I dropped to my knees imagining Craig standing invisible before me as I put my arms out to hug him. I visualised him in my arms and I told him over and over again that I loved him so much. I knelt there for a couple of minutes before standing and kissing Craig goodbye and finishing the cleaning.

I decided that I wasn't going to say anything to Barbara about any of this. She was already finding it difficult to hold on to her belief that Craig had been communicating with us at all. In her darkest moments she reasoned that all the occurrences could have been merely coincidental, and of course she could be right. None of what happened to us could ever be constituted as proof, by any stretch of the imagination. Barbara was far less open to these experiences than I was, that's for sure. So I decided there was no point in saying anything.

However, the next day we were driving from Inch to Gorey on our way back from lunch in Toss Byrne's. We were taking the scenic route when out of nowhere Barbara decided to share something with me. She told me that the previous day, while she was in the shower, she had become convinced that she'd heard Craig calling her name and felt that he was standing outside watching her. So utterly sure was she, that she simply had to get out of the shower and walk into the bedroom to see if he was there. She said how she literally could feel his presence in the room. When she told me this I was gobsmacked. I immediately told her about my experience, which obviously happened at the exact same moment that Barbara had hers. We were both tingling with the certainty that we had actually felt him around us. It was an extraordinary confirmation that our Craig had been in our presence and that we had felt him. When I thought back on how strong that pull on my sweater was, it lightened my heart and opened my mind to the connection that can be 'felt' across the divide. It showed me just how amazing our wonderful Craig is—to bridge that gap.

I Don't Need a Picture, To Remind Me of You . . .

I cannot recall the exact date of this communication but it was another powerful example of how Craig came back to help heal our broken hearts. We were having another really bad day. Barbara more so in fact. She was in a very dark place in her mind and was crying her heart out to me about not being able to carry on without Craig. I was trying my best to bring any form of comfort that I could, but I knew it was something that Barbara just had to 'feel' and that there was nothing I could do to change or remove the pain she felt in her soul. We were sitting together on the couch in the sitting room, Barbara crying and me listening, and talking about those more difficult memories that we experienced towards the end of Craig's life.

Barbara simply couldn't stop playing them over and over in her mind and they were tormenting her. She felt that Craig was so hard done by—as were we for losing him—and the pain, that evening, was too much for her to suppress. As we sat there in darkest misery we heard an almighty crash. We both actually jumped in our seats. We turned to look behind us to where the noise had come from. What we saw sent our heart rates racing. Just behind the couch, against the wall, we had a large press covered in many picture frames and ornaments. When we looked at it, one of the larger picture frames had fallen over. I got up and walked over to check it out. This large picture frame, which was completely surrounded by many other smaller ones, and various ornamental figures, was lying 'face down' in its spot. It had fallen down without disturbing a single thing around it. The natural leaning angle of the frame would have made it impossible to fall over into this position and certainly not without disturbing the other bits and pieces around it. It was extraordinary. When I lifted the frame it showed a picture of Craig being hugged by his mammy. We both knew that this was another sign. The noise, the nature and the timing of this falling picture told us both that Craig was again letting us know that he was here with us.

On two other occasions, many months after this one, and many months apart, a similar communication from Craig was sent. On the first of these occasions, we were again in the sitting room and we were both having a tough time. We were being very emotional about Craig when we heard another horrendous bang. We looked over to the corner of the room where the noise had come from and were amazed to see that a picture of Craig was lying down in the midst of other tightly packed picture frames. Like in the first instance it had fallen face down and without disturbing anything else around it. On the next occasion, Barbara and I were lying in our bed in the early hours of the morning (perhaps 2 a.m. or so) reminiscing about Craig and crying, when all of a sudden we heard a loud bang coming from downstairs. We were absolutely terrified. We were convinced that a burglar had got into the house and had most likely dropped something.

I cautiously came down the stairs and checked out the whole place. Nothing! I turned on all the lights and checked every room. I even went outside to check out there. Again nothing. It was only when I was turning off the last light in the sitting room that I happened to glance over at the press at the opposite wall. My heart leapt as I saw a picture lying face down in among the others. It was a picture of Craig and like the others hadn't disturbed anything else around it. My lips and chin shook as I stared at the picture and thanked Craig for coming back to us like this. I placed the frame neatly back and ran upstairs to tell Barbara. We just hugged each other and thanked Craig again for being such an extraordinary, wonderful son. We slept peacefully after that. It seemed as if Craig always came to us when we were in the depths of despair and chose those times as we needed it most.

Testimony of Light . . .

A number of months passed before we next received a message from Craig. It was 2 July 2007 and on this occasion it happened as I entered my office/spare room. I had been downstairs when I heard Barbara calling me, so ran up to see what the matter was. She was in our room cleaning and putting away clothes when she found a book that belonged to me in one of her drawers. She wanted me to put it away in my own room with the rest of the others.

When I saw the book she had found I was delighted. It was one that I'd misplaced months earlier and actually thought that I'd lost. Neither of us had any idea how it came to be in Barbara's drawer but I took it anyway and walked into my room to put it away. As I did I reached out to switch on the light. As soon as I flicked the switch the light above me began to strobe like nothing I'd ever seen before. I stood motionless as I watched the strange pulsing light and contemplated whether this was yet another communication from Craig.

I started to speak out, saying 'I know it's you, Craig. I know it's you, darlin',' when it occurred to me that Barbara was only in the next room and would want to see this. I shouted for her to come in and when she stood and watched the strange pulsing she was overcome. As we stood transfixed I began telling Barbara what had happened and as I gestured towards the pulsing light with my left hand I noticed the title of the book that was being held aloft—*Testimony of Light*—*Proof of Life after Death*. I couldn't believe how relevant it was. Craig's lightshow was certainly a testimony to his survival of what we call death.

Barbara then asked me whether I had my phone with me, to video it. I checked my pocket and found it. I recorded the light pulsing away and showed the book, with its title, in my hand. I still have that recording, saved onto my laptop.

In January 2009 that very same pulsing light effect happened again but this time in the upstairs bathroom. I was downstairs in the kitchen when I heard Barbara calling for me. It was evening time and dark outside, so when I came out to the hall to make my way upstairs to Barbara I was startled to see the dark hallway flashing with a light that was clearly coming from upstairs. I ran up to see what was going on and just when I got to the top of the landing I turned to see Barbara standing in the bathroom doorway, looking up at the pulsating light within. I couldn't believe it was happening again. We both stood and watched, basking in the presence of our Craig, knowing that the signal was coming from him. We spoke with him and hoped that he could hear our every word.

Mr Mischief...

On 26 May 2007 we attended a memorial mass in Crumlin Children's Hospital for all the children who had passed away. It was a very emotional time for us. In addition to the ceremony we were also being permitted to see Craig's name and details which had been added to a large book that Crumlin kept for all its deceased children. It was devastating to see Craig's name listed in among the countless other dead children's names and was something that my father couldn't even bear to look at. He could only cry for Craig and watch us bear witness to this dreaded book from the other side of the church.

But it was during the prior memorial service that something curious happened; something which we like to think was the activity of our mischievous little Craig. It was during a section of the service when all the parents or guardians were asked to come up and light candles for their loved ones. It was tragic to see such a long queue but up we went awaiting our turn. When it came to my turn I received the lit candle from the priest and turned to bring it to the altar where it was to be placed with the others. As I approached the altar the flame blew out. I turned back around quickly to the priest and asked him to relight the candle which he did. I carefully turned around and began again, but watched in horror as the flame once again just 'blew out'. In a moment of complete awkwardness, and fully aware that I was now holding up the queue, I reached back to the priest and politely, and apologetically, asked if he could please light it once again. He did, and this time I walked as slowly as I could to the altar.

I couldn't actually believe my eyes as the candle 'blew out' again just as I began to place it down on the altar. *For fuck sake*, I thought to myself as I shook my head in disbelief.

'It's being stubborn, is it?' asked a lady who was standing at the altar, before reaching out with an extended candle stick thingy—complete with roaring flame—and relighting my candle.

'Thanks,' I said, smiling briefly as I turned to walk away and watched with astonishment (and fury) as my candle once again 'blew out'. I returned to my seat defeated and looked up at the altar filled with dozens of lit candles, all surrounding my 'stubbornly' unlit loner. I was actually feeling despair that my candle for Craig was sitting up there extinguished. Barbara came back to her seat at that point and I whispered to her what happened and how upset I was that my candle was up there without any flame. I was upset for Craig.

'That was Craig blowing it out,' Barbara said instantly.

It had never occurred to me, but as soon as Barbara said it, I felt wonderful. And it was exactly the kind of thing that Craig would do. I was a sitting duck and he got me good! I fell for it hook, line and sinker. I delighted in thinking of him, watching, giggling at me—his victim—as I fumbled in such an awkward and emotionally charged situation. I was like a mouse in his cat claws. It was brilliant. Then Barbara told me that her candle just wouldn't light at all and she had to leave it on the altar unlit too. I looked up at the altar and could see our two candles standing out a mile. It was incredible to think that our boy had come to us yet again, and in such playful mood, at such a difficult time for us.

Wouldn't Miss It for the World

It was Barbara's fortieth birthday on 9 January 2009. This was always going to be a mixed affair for Barbara. Turning forty is bad enough but Barbara had always planned to have a party to 'celebrate' it rather than be miserable. In fact, it was something that she spoke about and planned years before and a party that Craig would always ask about. Barbara remembers how excited Craig became when after asking 'Can I go to it?' she'd replied, 'Of course you can!' He was ecstatic, with his energy levels flying into overdrive. Barbara said that he could stay up late and hang around with all of us adults—words that were the sweetest music to Craig's ears.

Over the years Craig would frequently bring up the 'party', completely out of the blue. He just wanted Barbara to talk about it so he could indulge his excitement over and over again. It is no understatement to say that he simply couldn't wait. He'd always loved birthday parties—although he didn't always get one—so this was going to be a big one.

Barbara was initially reluctant to do anything for her fortieth after Craig passed away. She felt that it just wasn't right or that she didn't have the energy for it. I knew exactly where she was coming from but

I also knew how sociable Barbara was and how much she 'needed' something like this. I asked her to reconsider. I said Craig would like nothing more than to see that party go ahead and that he would be there without any shadow of a doubt. He wouldn't like to see his mammy so unhappy on such a special occasion and he would probably send her a beautiful birthday message.

When I finally convinced Barbara to go ahead with it I suggested that the cabin in the Wicklow Mountains might be a good spot for having a get-together. We hired out the cabin for three days, from 11 to 13 January, with the party scheduled for the twelfth. Barbara and I had also decided to get engaged for her birthday. This was my 'birthday present' to Barbara.

We decided to mark the ninth—Barbara's actual birthday and our official engagement date—by staying the night in the Talbot Hotel in Wexford. We wanted this to be our own private celebration and mark the actual day properly. We arrived early that afternoon and checked into our room. And it was a lovely room too. Before we left for a bit of browsing around the town we put a bottle of champagne aside to chill for our return: we intended to start the celebrations early that evening.

After a little saunter around we decided to go for a drink in White's Hotel. We sat down and ordered our drinks and looked out as the busy main street of Wexford was alive with people all out and about doing their thing. As we sat there, the room suddenly went dark. Silence and shadows gripped the room. We looked around us and could see the bar staff looking perplexed. In the next moment the lights came back on and the music returned. But even with the electricity restored, all the lights and wall lamps kept flickering on and off. Barbara and I looked at each other and wondered.

After we finished our first drink we decided on another, with Barbara making the order. Then, while at the bar all the electricity went yet again. Barbara looked back at me with a two eyebrow salute, pondering the significance of all that was happening. She returned after making the order and just as she sat down we watched as the electricity came back on again. Again the lights and lamps just kept flickering on and off and this time we believed it was Craig—I recognised his work.

'He's saying Happy Birthday to you,' I said to Barbara, as we both raised our glasses and said thanks to him.

Just then the Manager came down with our drinks and apologised for the problems with the electricity. I asked him what was going on but he said he didn't have a clue. He said that their electricity feed kept dropping out but nobody else on the street was affected. 'Normally,' he said, 'other shops on the street go down too, but for some reason the problem is only affecting us!' He even went on to say that the generator wasn't working right either and that was why, he reckoned, the lights were going up and down as they were. Barbara and I looked at each other, knowingly, before politely agreeing with the concerned and troubled Manager. We tipped our glasses to Craig again, wearing a smile on our lips and feeling the weight in our hearts. What a boy!

But the story didn't end there either, although we didn't realise it until many weeks after. You see, there was another twist; something that was only realised in retrospect. But I'll come back to that later. . .

The Atmosphere was Electric . . .

It seems Craig's preferred method of message sending is definitely electrical. I've already mentioned some examples above but there have been many such 'electrical incidents' which have followed us.

We've been away a handful of times to Edinburgh in the last couple of years and nearly every time we've been there we've run into some of these electrical issues. The first time, we had been out all day shopping and wandering about and had finally come back, turning the light on as we entered. As soon as we did, the lights flashed and we were left in complete darkness. I had to hold the door open to let the light from the corridor flood the room so we could see what we were doing. We rang down to the desk and told them about the problem. In a matter of minutes a man came to the room and checked a box that was over the door. 'The switch was tripped,' he said. 'Did you have a kettle, maybe a hairdryer or shower on at the same time?' he asked. We explained how we'd just walked into the room and turned the light on. He looked a little surprised at this before quietly leaving us. But Barbara and I wondered if it was our little man. We had asked him to let us know he was with us—if he could—while we were away. *Maybe he just had.*

A few months after this we were in Edinburgh again. On one of the nights we were there, Barbara awoke during the night to go to the toilet. As soon as she turned the bathroom light on, it blew, and all the electricity was gone from the room. We had to wait until morning to get the staff to fix it. At this point we felt coincidence was not an option and this *was* Craig saying 'Hello'.

Some months, perhaps a year after this, we were in Edinburgh again and were staying at the Royal British Hotel. We had managed to fluke the top 'suite' room in the hotel, after only booking a basic double room. We didn't question it, but certainly enjoyed it. On the first night we were there we were shaken out of our beds by an extremely loud internal fire alarm. The noise was deafening. It was about 5 a.m. and we jumped out of the bed and got dressed as quickly as we could. We figured the whole hotel would be evacuated as a precaution so, nursing hangovers, we were rushing around like idiots, throwing clothes on. Just as we were fully dressed, the alarm stopped. *Typical*, we thought. I rang down to reception and asked what the problem had been. The receptionist said he didn't know what had caused it, but it may be something to do with the kitchens. *At 5 a.m. in the morning*, I thought, but said nothing. Barbara and I recognised immediately Craig's now familiar handy work and told him he was a *divil*—and that we loved him for it.

The following brief accounts represent, not a direct experience of ours, but rather accounts passed on to us by others. I'll begin with something that was shared with us by Barbara's brother Shane . . .

Little Minds at Play

Barbara received a text from Shane on 18 October 2007 relaying something which had happened that he wanted Barbara to know about. He told her how his own son, little Shane (who was about five at the time), had come up to him in the garden whilst playing on a toy mobile phone. Out of nowhere little Shane turned and said, 'Craig said that Peter fell off his bike.'

Shane and his wife Tracey couldn't believe what they heard. Their shock came from knowing that Peter (Barbara and Shane's younger brother), who tragically died in a drowning tragedy, had actually drowned in the river Boro after falling off his bike. Little Shane just wouldn't have known this at the time, and for him to have said it so out of the blue, so out of context, and to further attribute his knowing of that very fact to Craig telling him, was utterly astonishing. This is why Shane felt so compelled to tell Barbara about it. He just couldn't keep it to himself.

He also decided to tell us then of another time when little Shane came running into the sitting room one night, out from his bedroom, to collect a yellow car. 'Craig likes to play with the yellow one,' is all he said before returning to his room.

Invincible Friend

One day while we were out and about in Gorey we bumped into the mother of a school friend of Craig's. We spoke at length and in the course of this conversation we mentioned how we've had strange things happen in the house that we knew were messages from Craig. When we said this we were surprised to see this woman open up to us. She told us that her son still had a picture of Craig in his room and that she often overheard him in the room talking to Craig, as if he was in the room with him. I was delighted; more evidence of Craig's remarkable, invincible spirit.

––––

Before I finish this chapter I'd like to share one more example of how Craig has communicated with us from where he is. The reason I'm leaving this until the end is because of the timing of the communication. You see, the message came on the very day that I started to write this particular chapter. Craig is a clever boy. Given the potential for all his communications to be rationalised into complete dismissals, he often marries the timing of their delivery to a significant moment or situation. It is the coupling of these factors that strengthens our belief in the power and the impact of these messages from Craig.

In this last message Barbara and I, along with Dean who was sitting in his bouncer, were sitting watching the TV very late one evening on

5 April 2009. Dean was very restless and he had a terrible cough and cold. We had decided to stay up late until he fell asleep before bringing him up to bed and so were just vegging in front of the TV until the moment was right. As we sat there, the lamp in the corner of the room, which was behind us, began to flicker on and off. We both turned around to look at it and then looked at each other. The other lamp hadn't flickered at all. Neither of us said anything to each other. *Maybe it was just the bulb itself, who knows.* After a little while Barbara decided to bring Dean to bed and was so tired herself that she decided to put the head down too.

While she was upstairs I decided to lock up only to realise I needed to make one more bottle for Dean. I headed out to the kitchen and boiled the kettle while getting his powdered milk and sterilised bottle ready. As I was doing this the light overhead began to flicker. I looked up, and of the three bulbs that made up the light fixture, one was flickering on and off. When I saw this, and remembering the flickering lamp a little earlier, I truly believed it was Craig.

'I love you, Craig,' I said instantly. 'I love you and I miss you so much. I hope to God you're ok, Spud, and that you're happy.' Just then the light stopped flickering and resumed its normal operation. I smiled and turned around to make up the bottle.

When I finally went to bed I didn't say anything to Barbara who, I assumed, may have been asleep already. I climbed into the bed and within a few minutes I fell asleep. It was just before midnight. At 2 a.m. however I woke up to hear Dean farting in his cot and Barbara crying into her pillow. She told me that she couldn't stop thinking of Craig and that her heart was broken remembering all that he went through. We talked for a while as I tried to ask Barbara not to dwell on all the bad stuff but try and focus on the wonderful memories we had of him.

I had to say this, but I knew the place where Barbara was in her mind. No amount of reassurance or positivity could affect her state of mind then. It was that dark, festering hole of a place where those horrid memories simply would not be denied and where the mind had lost all grip on hope. I knew that place well and I knew no amount of words from me, or anyone, could have effected any change in Barbara's pain at that moment.

As we spoke, though, Barbara told me that while she had been lying there the light from the bathroom (which we always left on so as to flood our room with some gentle light for Dean in his cot) had started to flicker on and off. It was then that I told Barbara what happened downstairs just before I came up to bed. We were convinced then that it must be Craig reassuring us he was still around, trying to comfort us in our despair. Then, right on cue, the light from the bathroom began to flicker on and off once again.

'Is that you, darlin'?' we both whispered out to the hall. 'We love you, Craig . . . we love you so much,' we called, and then the light stopped. At that moment, it dawned on me how I had just started this very chapter earlier that day—'The boy who lives'—so I told Barbara. He had chosen his moment wisely as always. All these factors—individual, separate bulbs flashing on and off around the house; the relevance of the chapter I was writing—coalesced to scream out loud that our beautiful Craig had come home for a visit.

Barbara fell asleep straight after that and it was I who lay there contemplating this extraordinary bridging of two worlds—this tenuous seam which simultaneously joins and parts truth from the unknown, and a family from being one.

———

But in death, as in life, Craig has proven to be an unstoppable force that has reached through the divide and shown us that his spirit is burning bright and will always do so. His fierce spirit, who all could see when he was here, pulled gently aside the veil between our worlds and allowed us a glimpse of truth. He has shown us that life and death, as we see it, is an illusion; that there is neither one nor the other, just a continuous but ever winding journey. A journey that we all share but one in which, for us, Craig has gone a little further on up the road. In his brief life and in his dying, Craig has shown us more about truth than anyone or anything else and helped to catapult us on to a new path towards greater understanding.

He has shown me, by his example, how I should seek to live my life. In his honesty, in his wit, in his happiness, in his kindness, in his sense of justice and fair play, in his lovable mischief, in his tolerance, in his outrageous generosity of spirit, in the uncompromising freedom of his expression and in his courage in the face of all that would pull him down he gave a true masterclass in how life is to be lived and showed me and his mammy, and in various degrees all who knew him, that life is to be lived and how best to do it.

Chapter 11

New Beginnings

The grieving process is a painful one: a lifetime in shadow for those parents who've lost a child. I've heard it remarked that losing a child is the single most painful thing that any human can go through in a lifetime. Barbara and I certainly couldn't disagree. It is an exquisite, indefinite excruciation of the mind and soul which tears apart all that you know to be real and worthwhile and leaves you like some raddled castaway lost to an infinite oblivion. It is hell.

When your child dies, you occupy a world where only you exist now. Nobody else lives where you live. Nobody else sees or feels what you do. Even your partner, who shares the very same loss as you, inhabits his/her own private world of suffering and confusion. You are united by a common love and a common loss but your paths of personal understanding, contemplation, adaptation, acceptance, progression and healing can only ever be yours alone to walk. You must find your own way along that meandering trail that leads always *away* from your past—that which you knew and hold dear—and on to some unknown existence. It is the fear of this unknown and the separation from your beloved past that is the scourge of your new life.

Everyone grieves differently, they say, and I can only speak now with experience, not expertise. There are enough experts out there who can agree or disagree with anything I have to say on the topic of parental grief. It's really not important to me or to Barbara. What we feel is neither right nor wrong, it merely *is*, and our journey and our experiences both individually and together are all we can speak of.

When Craig died, neither I nor Barbara ever sought counselling or any kind of professional help in dealing with our grief. We just lived through it. We've never really bent the ears of our friends or families about our pain. We have largely kept it to ourselves. And yes, we both continue to speak of Craig whenever we feel like it, remembering all the great things he did and said but we've never confided in another the depths of our pain and the despair that has ruined our lives. We've never burdened anyone with our 'baggage'. I guess we've always felt that nobody really wants to hear it. Sometimes when we have, it's amazing actually to see how some people just try to change the subject or dilute it with some misplaced positivity that neither applies nor helps and in fact only infuriates. I guess people do not want to see it. They're afraid of it. And in all honesty I would be too, I suppose. So Barbara and I have just gone about our lives quietly and with our social masks at the ready at all times.

But even Barbara and I are very different in how we handle our grief. Our coping mechanisms, our expectations and our needs are poles apart on so many different levels. For example, I am much more detached and therefore largely unaffected by the insensitivity of others. I'm not sure whether this is necessarily a good thing as it may simply highlight my own emotional, or perhaps more accurately, social inadequacies. Those inadequacies may only come into their own in situations like this, but I guess largely leave other areas of my life so much the poorer. In any case, it makes our grieving all the more different.

One significant area where Barbara and I differed only became apparent within a few months of Craig passing away. Barbara brought up the subject of having a baby and it just wasn't something that was even on my radar. I actually couldn't stomach the idea of having another child. When Craig had died one of the things I remember struggling with was my new sense of identity. I had always been comfortable with being a family man. I loved it. When Craig died, though, we were thrown back into just being a couple and I hated it. But, even so, the suggestion of having another baby was something I just didn't even want to think about.

Every last drop of my emotions were for Craig. All I could think of was what I could do to learn more about the true nature of this world we live in and spend my life trying to find him. I felt that having another child was like turning my back on him and represented some kind of acceptance that I neither had nor indeed wanted. I did not want another child. I wanted Craig.

But I appreciated Barbara's position, our position. Barbara didn't want to have a child then either, but she was 39 and I suppose we just didn't have time to wait. I was approaching 31 and it was the first time that the age gap became an issue with us. I was so annoyed that Barbara was that age and that we had this extra burden on our shoulders to deal with. I wasn't angry with Barbara, just the situation. Everything in me said I wasn't in a place to do this but still we pressed on.

We tried for a number of months without success and it was so incredibly stressful. One day Barbara and I decided to go to Wexford Town, just to get out of the house. As we made our way down the main street Barbara told me that she was a little overdue, menstrually speaking that is, and the more she spoke the more she began to tie herself in knots of anxiety. Walking along we passed a Superdrug store so I stopped. 'Right,' I said. 'Let's just go in and get the bloody pregnancy test and stop all this himmin' and hawwin' about mights and maybes. Let's get the test and see what is the situation.' I didn't want to have to listen to Barbara's anxiety for the next five or six days when there was no need.

So, in we went. We looked around all the shelves but couldn't find any of the tests. We were being super cautious too. It's amazing really, but here we were, two grown adults skulking around the back aisles trying to disguise the fact that we were looking for a pregnancy test. We actually hadn't told anyone that we were trying for a baby so there was an element of fear that someone might walk into the chemist's and see us—with IT in our hands.

But try as we might we couldn't find any. 'Can I help you there?' asked one of the staff, the volume ear-shatteringly loud—to us anyway.

'Emm,' we began, quietly, hoping to set the tone, 'we're looking for your pregnancy tests. We can't find them.'

The lady walked us over to a section where she believed them to be and was surprised when there were none there. But not as surprised as we were as she then proceeded to almost burst her larynx in shouting to the front of the shop, 'Mary! . . . Where do we keep the pregnancy tests?'—the whole queue now looking back in our direction, and a passer-by outside too. It was actually very funny. We just laughed at each other and eventually bought one—the circumstance of its purchase now an anecdote for the future.

Later that evening when we were home I was upstairs working at the computer when Barbara came into the room behind me. The first thing that struck me were the words 'I'm pregnant.'

I turned around, looking at Barbara and then down at the two blue lines that were displayed on the tester in her hand.

'We're going to have a baby,' she reaffirmed with emotion and shock in her voice.

And it certainly was a shock to me. I stood up and hugged her and felt a curious mixture of excitement, relief and deepest sadness. Our eyes welled up as we walked straight into Craig's room to tell him the news. With tears we began telling him that he was going to have a baby brother or sister. We sat on his bed and talked to him, and in our hearts we cried for the family that we should have been. We cried for our Craig: cried that he would never get to know his brother or sister and never be a part of our lives as we would surely grow as a family together. We cried for our baby who would never get to know his wonderful big brother. There was such terrible pain in the scale of the loss.

But the fusion of emotions was strong and our excitement grew slowly. It was an emergent joy that brimmed and bubbled gently to the surface. It was such an incredible feeling to know that we would be parents again; that we'd have a little baby to look after and to love. It truly felt like we'd been blessed with another life, and although it was wrought with such incredible pain, we embraced and absorbed this beautiful gift and thanked the heavens for what it gave.

As we lay in the bed that night talking and thinking, it suddenly dawned on Barbara that she must have been pregnant when she'd had her fortieth birthday up in the cabin. We tried to think back to when the baby was conceived. I remember feeling an extraordinary shiver down my spine as I realised the probable date: it was actually on the calendar day of Barbara's fortieth birthday. It had been the night we'd stayed in Wexford. The significance began to sink in: on that day Barbara turned forty; we became officially engaged; Barbara got pregnant and Craig had come to say Happy Birthday to his mammy while we were in White's Hotel having a drink. All this happened on the same day. It was extraordinary. The timing was just phenomenal. It was a beautiful feeling for us to believe that Craig may have had a hand in it all. Later, in fact, when we told people about the pregnancy both Barbara's mother and mine revealed that they had had dreams around the time of Barbara's birthday in which Craig came to them and said, 'My mammy's going to have a baby.' It was incredible. All this restored our connectedness and allowed us to relax in Craig's continuing presence in our lives. It made us feel like he was giving us his personal blessing to move on with our lives and also that he was showing us, yet again, that he was and always would be with us wherever and whenever that may be. It was a warm feeling.

———

On 24 September 2008, at exactly 2.05 a.m., we were blessed with a beautiful baby boy—Dean. He was 8 lb 10 oz and perfect. Lying on Barbara's chest we both stared into his beautifully wrinkled, Mr Magoo head and thanked the heavens for his safe delivery.

He was our little miracle. We touched his little hands and rubbed his little face and we stared at each other. It was a happiness that I cannot relay. Dean was the most sacred gift to us and we felt so proud and happy. The feeling of love that coursed through our veins was incredible. We held him protectively and stroked him all over. We kissed his little head over and over again and told him how much we loved him. It was this tactile expression of our love that we'd gone so long without and so we drank it up—every last drop. The physical bonding was intoxicating and the joy that filled our hearts was powerful. It was an incredible moment for us both—to hold a child in our arms once more.

For all the joy that we felt in that moment, there was always going to be such sadness too. Our thoughts turned to Craig and how happy he'd have been to see his little brother. He'd always wanted a baby brother or sister—he'd told us so on many occasions, saying something like, 'Why can't I have a brother or sister? It's not fair. Everyone else I know has one . . .'

So having Dean also brought with it that measure of sorrow. Also, knowing Dean would grow up not knowing his brother and perhaps, if we let it, suffer a life of being in Craig's shadow. We wouldn't allow this, of course, but then you never can tell. We'd probably never fully understand how Dean would react to living with the ghost of his unknown brother, and a past that he was never part of.

Craig and Dean: two brothers who never met, who never would meet in this life and who were both robbed of a life of close brotherhood and the joys and laughter that surely would have been theirs.

But we also knew that Craig *was* around us in some way and that he would always be part of our family here. We had to hold on to the belief that our entire family was united in some unseen way and though the physicality of Craig's absence was so impossible to bear, his life force surrounded us all and bathed us in his love, his light and his wonderful, unconquerable spirit. He would always, always be with us.

But the beauty, the treasure and the salvation that is Dean filled our souls with such immeasurable joy. It was the essence of hope, of love and of deepest gratitude for him coming into our lives. He was only seconds old and we loved him so. The moment, the reality of having him here with us just then, was so overwhelmingly beautiful that we simply kept smiling.

When Dean was allowed to leave the hospital the first place we headed for was Craig's grave. It was very emotional for Barbara and me to be there with our two sons, worlds apart from each other, but bonded by love. The body of our firstborn, Craig, lay deep in the cold earth and that of Dean's in the warmth of our arms. Such contrasting feelings: pain and love, hope and loss, life and death. There were moments of silence between us then. We both allowed each other space to be in the moment and to share our private thoughts, our tears and our quiet words with our beloved Craig and to tell him that he had gotten his wish of being a big brother. We whispered into our beautiful little Dean's ears and told him of how special he was and how lucky we were to have been blessed with two beautiful boys. We vowed to tell him all about his big brother and shared with him our belief that Craig would look out for him all his days. We stayed there for a while until we finally took Dean to see his home.

Walking through that door and bringing a new life into the house was a special moment. It was like a window opening into a blackened, deserted building, spreading sunshine and breezes into its every darkened corner. We looked down at the tiny little bundle that lay sleeping at our feet and we felt love. We reflected on the time when we had first brought Craig home and remembered our initial apprehension and awe. But with Dean it was very different. We looked upon this little miracle and instead of feeling nervous and unsure, we felt immense assuredness and a strong sense of purpose. We were his parents and we would do everything in our power to safeguard his beautiful precious life and to shower him with our love. We no longer took life for granted and our glorious little Dean was our promise of a future that we'd long since given up on.

At the time of writing this chapter Dean is nine months old. He is a beautiful, happy and healthy baby and the peace and joy that he has brought into our lives once again is a miracle that we are so deeply grateful for. Just his very presence in our lives has changed everything.

There is no denying the fact that he and Craig are so physically alike and that sometimes when he looks at us we can see his brother staring back. The resemblance will always be there. But Dean is very much Dean—nobody else. Already his personality is shining through and he is most definitely putting his own personal stamp on the world. He is beautiful and confident. He is wild and bustling with adventure. He is musical and mischievous. All these things we can see and feel as we live each day with him, basking in the love and hope that he brings.

He's too young to know it now of course but in time, we hope, he can begin to understand how imponderably precious his coming into our life has been. And not as some replacement for Craig or some salve for our wounds. No. Dean is *not* those things. The very notion is pre-posterous. Dean is a beautiful individual. He is our son. We love him for who he is, *because* he is. Just having him in our lives, to love and to guide, has been the greatest blessing. We cover him in kisses and hold him in our arms for the gorgeous little boy that he is and because we feel so lucky to have been gifted him.

In writing this book it is also my hope that in years to come, when Dean is older, he can one day pick it up and read about the brother he never knew. I hope that the true element of Craig's nature has been captured, even if only slightly, within these pages and that moments of his life can be glimpsed. Dean can of course never truly know Craig in this lifetime; they were both denied this right. I just hope that the book, along with all of our pictures and videos, and through the stories we will certainly tell can go some way to bridging the divide and bring them closer. They deserve it.

——

Throughout the writing of this book Barbara found it impossible to really get involved. I asked her to write down or recount her memories of Craig so that I could add them in, but she just wasn't able. The pain was too much. So inevitably the book reads largely from my perspective. There was no avoiding this. But Barbara did manage to put a small note together and I want to add this here now and so let her voice be heard:

I could write so many stories about my darling Craig and each are equally wonderful. As a mother of two beautiful boys it's sad to know that they never met in this life. I will try and give Dean a wonderful life full of love and happiness and one day I'll explain the loss his mammy and daddy felt over his brother. This book will be his to cherish too so that he can read about and get to know his brother a little. But I'll also tell Dean how his coming into our lives gave us such hope and reason to live on . . . that he saved our lives.

   When I think of dying, when I dream of heaven, I see Craig as the six-year-old boy that I know, standing there waiting to meet me. And he will see me like he remembers, not like some old lady—if I get to that age. I dream of hearing him calling out 'Mammy' once more, and then catching my hand as he always did. That is the dream that I hold in my heart for when my time comes to pass. I hope it will come true.

And so now, Craig, we finally speak to you directly. We both want to say something, but we won't keep you. I'll let your mammy speak first . . .

Dearest Craig,
My memories of you—how could I ever forget? You were so special to me. My son; my very bestest friend. Life without you is so hard, my darlin'. That song: 'Oh My Darlin', do you remember? Remember how I used to sing it to you when you were sick and you'd be in beside me in the bed? Or 'You are my sunshine'—how I'd sing that so softly while you were in my arms. You used to hold my neck so tight that I could hardly breathe. I was always afraid that you were so scared even though you never let on. You would always say 'I'll never leave you, Mammy.'

'I love you, Mammy'—How hard it is not to hear you say that anymore. The day you died, Craig—that morning—do you remember how I needed to go to the toilet and how I told you I'd be back in a minute and that Daddy would stay with you. You opened your eyes and followed me to the bathroom. You were saying goodbye to me. You closed your eyes and then never opened them again. My regret, Craig, is that I should have climbed straight back into bed with you and held you, telling you how much I love you and that everything would be fine.

I have to live with this and I'm so sorry. But I love you, my Craig. You know that. My love for you will go on forever and I know that we will be together again. I dream of that time always and I want you to know how happy you made my life. I thank you for loving me and letting me love you back.

My beautiful and very special little darling—I love you.

Mammy

——

Craig,
You know how difficult it has been to write this book. You've no doubt watched me cry, blubber and snot my way through endless hours of it. At times I've certainly felt you around me. I'm pretty certain the book will be found wanting but it is the best I could do, Spud. I just wanted people to know you were here; that you lived, that you loved and were loved by many. I wanted them to hear about the boy who made us all smile; who with charm, wit and intellect shone a most luminous light into the darkness of our world and changed it forever. I wanted them to sample even the tiniest bit of the might of you.

Craig, darlin', you have defined my life. From the first whispers of your arrival to the screaming tears of your bitter parting you stormed into my world and breathed purpose and meaning into it. You revolutionised my existence and I thank you for choosing us, being with us and for the legacy of the beautiful memories you have left with us.

I think of you all the time. You are simply never absent from my thoughts. Even with the recent heavy snow I thought instantly of you, and what you'd do. That's why I stripped naked in the snow, danced wildly and made snow angels in the back garden that night. Your mother thought I'd lost it, but I did it for you.

In your death, Craig, you have shown me more about life than I knew possible. In reflecting on your life I have learned so much about living. In loving you and losing you I have experienced the purest emotions of my life. You have been my greatest teacher, my closest friend and the inspiration for a lifetime.

I love you, Craig. I miss you. But I will see you again . . .

Be happy, Spud!

My eternal love,
Daddy

PS. I know you were there to greet your little cousin, Corey James, whose time was so painfully brief here. Watch over him and mind each other. You're two very special boys for sure. I'd like to finish your book now with the poem I wrote for you, Craig.

Your Life

Perched atop a chestnut sprig, swaying soft in summer's breeze
Your breath of song escaped among the dancing living leaves
And up through dappled green and gold, a wisp unto the blue
It sang a song of sentiment, of merriment . . . of You
Of love, of cheer, of happiness, of sun and season's heat
Of scented bloom and warmest moon, a tune so light and sweet
That o'er the sound of woodland stream and hoot and caw and rush
It soared so high that heavens sighed and all just stood in hush
For your song was the sweetest song the wind had ever heard
Who carried it with rhetoric—from such a little bird!
And every ear that bent to hear the beauty of your song
Wallowed in its majesty; mellifluous and strong
But under-crush of sodden leaves; the cool and misty rain
The cloud-filled skies that darkened eyes began to hint at change
And still you perched atop that sprig and sang your merry song
So all who cried, though listening out, in reverence sang along
Then quietly and gently a snow began to fall
And though it pained your reddening breast, you still let out your call
But now beyond that icy perch in still of winter's freeze
Your breath of song sings ever strong—above the fallen leaves